REPORT OF MICHIGAN FRESH UNPROCESSED WHOLE MILK WORKGROUP

Presented to Director Jamie Clover Adams
Michigan Department of Agriculture and Rural Development
December 11, 2012

Foreword by Sally Fallon Morell

Skyhorse Publishing

Table of Contents

Foreword V

Preface xix

Report of Michigan Fresh Unprocessed Whole Milk Workgroup

Recommendations...2
Recommended Next Steps..3

About the Michigan Fresh Unprocessed Whole Milk Workgroup
Purpose, Goal and Background 4
Lists: Members and Invited Subject Matter Experts 6

Discussion Summaries 9

Topic 1 – History of Fresh Unprocessed Whole Milk 11

1. Historically, why is milk an important component of our diet? 13
2. What is the history of milk regulation?...14
3. Why is milk one of the most regulated foods in the U.S.? 16
4. Is there something uniquely hazardous about milk? 17
5. Initially, what were the conditions that prompted pasteurization
   for milk; have those conditions and knowledge/understanding
   changed today? 17
References 19

Topic 2 – Benefits and Values 21

1. What is the nutritional value of milk? 23
   Nutritional Components Listed on Nutrition Facts Label. 25
2. Going beyond the Nutrition Facts label, what other nutritional
   values should we be considering?...28
3. What are the additional benefits of milk fresh from the cow?.............31
4. What is the impact of pasteurization on the value of FUW milk? 37
   Table - Impact of Heat, Temperature, and Time 40
5. What is the impact of homogenization on FUW milk's value?.............44

6. Assuming that all milk is not the same, what do production and management practices have to do with FUW milk's nutritional value, pathogens, color, taste, etc.? 44
7. What is the impact of consumer preferences on production and management practices of FUW milk? 46
References 47

Topic 3 – Risks 51

Introduction
    1. What are the risks for fresh, unprocessed whole milk, including all types of risks, such as pathogens, adverse consequences, intolerance, and allergens?
    2. Where do these risks originate? 53
Milkborne Bacterial Human Pathogen Summaries
    Campylobacter jejuni...54
    Listeria monocytogenes..58
    Salmonella..64
    Escherichia coli..67
Sidebar – Lateral Transfer of Genetic Material 70
Sidebar – Differing Perspectives 71
References 73
Scenarios for Transmission
    Campylobacter jejuni...75
    Listeria monocytogenes 78
    Salmonella 82
    Escherichia coli..85
Discussion of Infectious Dose 90
Other pathogens of historical milk-related public health concerns 91
Categories of risk other than infectious disease for people consuming fresh unprocessed whole milk 95
Adverse Consequences Unique to Fresh Unprocessed Whole Milk Consumption 99
Table of Terms 100

Topic 4 – Risk and Benefit Management 113

Introduction
    1. What steps are necessary to minimize the health risk for
       consumers of fresh unprocessed whole milk?
    2. Who is responsible for minimizing risk, as it relates to
       fresh unprocessed whole milk? 115
Table of Risk Management 117
    Hygiene 117
    Consumer Preferences 118
    Dairy Animals 119
    Milk 122
    Monitoring, Laboratory Testing, and Record-keeping 124
    Sources of Pathogens Virulent in People 126
    Water 130
3. What steps can be taken to mitigate or prevent adverse impacts
    on the entire dairy industry in the event of a milkborne
    outbreak originating from milk consumption? 131
4. What management practices enhance benefits? 133
Table of Benefit Management 133

Topic 5 – Consumer Choice Options 137

1. How might consumer access to fresh unprocessed
    whole milk be achieved? 139
2. How might people who are considering choosing to drink fresh
    unprocessed whole milk be properly educated and informed on
    their choice? 139

Food Safety & Inspection Program 141

Afterword 143

Cited References 151

FOREWORD

Sally Fallon Morell

It was just 12 ago that herd share agreements for the distribution of raw milk became legal in the State of Michigan, thanks to the persevering efforts of Dr. Ted Beals, MD, and the Michigan Fresh Unprocessed Whole Milk Workgroup (Workgroup). Today, nearly 120 farmers supply raw milk to Michigan consumers through herd share agreements, including seven in the Upper Peninsula. These farms are distributed fairly evenly across the state, making raw milk convenient and accessible to the entire population. The citizens of Michigan—and especially the children whose parents are wise enough to bring their children up on nature's perfect food—owe a great debt of thanks to Dr. Beals, the principal author of the Report.

According to the U.S. Food and Drug Administration (FDA) and other health agencies, pasteurization of milk is the greatest public health initiative in the history of mankind. It was pasteurization that eliminated infectious illness in the U.S. and that protects us against foodborne illness today, they say. Raw milk is inherently dangerous, is the mantra, "and should not be consumed by anyone under any circumstances at any time for any reason." And since pasteurization does not diminish the health-giving properties of milk and has no undesirable effects in any way—"Research has shown that there is no significant difference in the nutritional value of pasteurized and unpasteurized milk," is the way they put it, why not? Why not make pasteurization mandatory and spend our tax dollars in efforts to prevent our citizens from obtaining raw milk?

These government claims are easily refuted, starting with the assertion that pasteurization laws were responsible for the decline in deaths from childhood illnesses. Lawmakers imposed the first statewide pasteurization laws in 1948— and this was in the state of Michigan. By this time, deaths from measles, scarlet fever, whooping cough, typhoid and diphtheria had fallen to almost zero, from highs of 40 per hundred thousand people for diphtheria and typhoid, and

Report of Michigan Fresh Unprocessed Whole Milk Workgroup

around 15 per hundred thousand for measles, scarlet fever and whooping cough in 1900.[1]

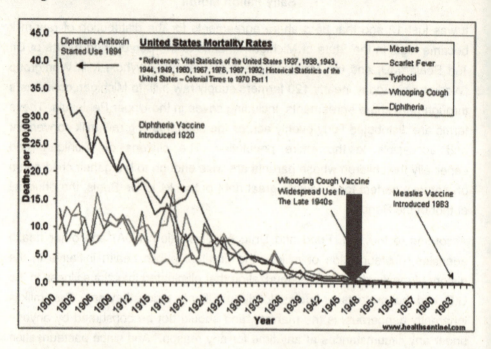

No one today would dispute the fact that these improvements were due to the installation of sewage systems and clean water supplies in the cities, and the elimination of piles of manure from city streets with the transition of horse-drawn transportation to the automobile. It was only in the early 1900s, for example, that the City of Chicago stopped drawing drinking water from the same area of Lake Michigan where sewage was dumped, and also began the chlorination of water supplies. After that, deaths from typhoid fever declined precipitously to zero in the mid-1940s, several years before mandatory pasteurization was ushered in.

And we know a lot more about milk today than we did during the push-for-pasteurization era. We know that milk contains numerous anti-microbial components that kill pathogens, strengthen the immune system, and help build a robust gut wall to prevent the passage of toxins. These include lactoferrin, lactoperoxidase, lymphocytes, immunoglobulins, antibodies, hormones and growth factors, mucins, fibronectin, glycomacropeptide, bifidus factor, B12-binding protein, lactoglobulins . . . the list of these beneficial, antimicrobial components grows with each year of research. Most are inactivated by pasteurization and all are destroyed by the very high heat of ultra-pasteurization.

Because of these components, raw milk passes the "challenge test," that is, when pathogens are added to raw milk, they do not multiply but gradually diminish to zero. Yes, raw milk kills pathogens! Pathogens added to pasteurized milk will multiply and grow, often morphing into super bugs that are hard to eliminate.

Many of these same components attach to nutrients in milk to facilitate their complete assimilation. Lactoferrin ensures that the iron in milk is 100% absorbed; B12 binding protein attaches to vitamin B12 and carries it across the gut wall; lactoglobulins perform the same task for vitamins A and D, and possibly other nutrients.

Raw milk is rich in cholesterol and contains several enzymes that ensure complete assimilation of the cholesterol. The infant needs cholesterol to build his brain, nervous system and gut wall, and for hormone production. Baby boys up to six months of age have (or are supposed to have) testosterone levels equal to those of an adult male. This priming ensures that he expresses male characteristics at puberty. Testosterone is made out of cholesterol, cholesterol the baby can't make at such a young age, but which he must absorb from milk. If the milk is pasteurized, the enzymes that help him do this will be destroyed. (There is no cholesterol at all in infant formula made from skim milk and vegetable oils.)

"Research has shown that there is no significant difference in the nutritional value of pasteurized and unpasteurized milk," say the bureaucrats, and this is technically true. If you measure the levels of calcium in raw and pasteurized

---

Report of Michigan Fresh Unprocessed Whole Milk Workgroup

milk, they will be the same. But how is the calcium being used? In 1940s experiments at Randleigh Farm, New York, researchers demonstrated that rats fed unpasteurized milk had longer bones, and much denser bones than rats fed pasteurized milk—because the calcium from unpasteurized is much more easily absorbed. The rats on pasteurized milk also showed signs of vitamin B6 deficiency.

The fact is, every nutrient in milk is compromised and often completely destroyed by heat treatment; the following table[2] describes the effect of pasteurization on some of these nutrients.

LOWERED NUTRIENT AVAILABILITY AFTER PASTEURIZATION

Vitamin C	Raw milk but not pasteurized can resolve scurvy. ". . . Without doubt. . . the explosive increase in infantile scurvy during the latter part of the 19th century coincided with the advent of use of heated milks. . ." [Rajakumar, Pediatrics. 2001;108(4):E76]
Calcium	Longer and denser bones on raw milk. [Studies from Randleigh Farms]
Folate	Carrier protein inactivated during pasteurization. [Gregory. J. Nutr. 1982, 1329-1338]
Vitamin B12	Binding protein inactivated by pasteurization.
Vitamin B6	Animal studies indicate B6 poorly absorbed from pasteurized milk. [Studies from Randleigh Farms]
Vitamin B2	Completely destroyed [*Journal of Food Protection* 74(11):1814-32]
Vitamin A	Beta-lactoglobulin, a heat-sensitive protein in milk, increases intestinal absorption of vitamin A. Heat degrades vitamin A. Said and others. [Am J Clin Nutr. 1989;49:690-694. Runge and Heger. J Agric Food Chem. 2000 Jan;48(1):47-55]
Vitamin D	Present in milk bound to lactoglobulins, pasteurization cuts assimilation in half. Hollis and others. [J Nutr. 1981;111:1240-1248; FEBS Journal 2009 2251-2265]

Iron	Lactoferrin, which contributes to iron assimilation, destroyed during pasteurization. Children on pasteurized milk tend toward anemia.
Minerals	Bound to proteins, inactivated by pasteurization; Lactobacilli, destroyed by pasteurization, enhance mineral absorption. [BJN 2000 84:S91-S98; MacDonald and others. 1985]

The Report discusses recent studies showing that children who grow up on raw milk have fewer allergies and rashes and lower rates of respiratory illness and asthma compared to children consuming pasteurized milk. But these are not the first investigations of raw milk health benefits. As early as the 1920s, researchers were studying the effects of raw milk versus pasteurized among children in Boston. Children getting raw milk compared to pasteurized had better weight gain, stronger teeth, better growth, and lower incidence of rickets, TB and diarrhea. "A larger use of certified [raw] milk in infant feeding should be encouraged by the medical profession," said one of the researchers.[3]

Animal experiments found that pasteurized milk feeding led to infertility in rats, as well as anemia and "irritable" behavior. Rats on pasteurized milk had compromised integrity of the internal organs – their insides were "mushy."

Guinea pigs on pasteurized milk had poor growth, muscle stiffness, emaciation and weakness; they died within one year. Autopsy revealed atrophied muscles streaked with calcification and calcium deposits under the skin, in the joints, heart, and other organs. Guinea pigs on raw whole milk had excellent growth and no abnormalities.

A 1941 study carried out at the West of Scotland Agricultural College at Auchincruive, looked at two groups, each of eight calves, for 90 days; one group was fed on raw milk, the other on pasteurized milk. All the animals in the raw milk group finished the trial without mortality. In the pasteurized milk group, two died before they were 30 days old, and a third died on day 92; that is, two days after the experiment ended. The remaining calves in the pasteurization

Report of Michigan Fresh Unprocessed Whole Milk Workgroup

group were in ill health at the end of the experiment, while all of the animals in the raw milk group were in excellent health.[4]

In 1943, Dr. Evelyn Sprawson of the London Hospital declared, ". . . In certain institutions, children who were brought up on raw milk . . . had perfect teeth and no decay. The result is so striking and unusual that it will undoubtedly be made the subject of further inquiry."[5]

Tragically, this inquiry never happened. In fact, soon after the dairy industry—or at least their friends in high places—began a campaign against their competition, whole raw milk produced on small farms and sold directly to the consumer was stopped. In May, 1945, an article titled "Raw Milk Can Kill" appeared in *Coronet Magazine*.[6] The seemingly factual article was about a town called Crossroads, USA, where many died from undulant fever, contracted from raw milk. But the whole story was made up; there was no town called Crossroads, USA, and no outbreak of undulant fever! Undaunted, the August, 1946, *Reader's Digest* repeated the false story about Crossroads, USA. Just two years later, with the opposition muzzled by the Crossroads propaganda, the State of Michigan passed the first state mandatory pasteurization laws.

Lies about raw milk have continued since the Crossroads story. For example, in a 2012 PowerPoint presentation by posted on the FDA website [no longer accessible at www.cfsan.fda.gov/~ear/milksafe] and referenced in legislative testimony, John F. Sheehan, former Director at the Division of Plant and Dairy Food Safety, contends that pasteurization is the only way to ensure the safety of milk. Sheehan cites fifteen studies claimed to link raw milk with illness; however, in a published rebuttal by the Weston A. Price Foundation,[7] scrutiny of the studies revealed the following:

No Valid Positive Milk Sample	12/15	80%
No Valid Statistical Association with Raw Milk	10/15	67%
Findings Misrepresented by FDA	7/15	47%
Alternatives Discovered, Not Pursued	5/15	33%
No Evidence Anyone Consumed Raw Milk Products	2/15	13%
Outbreak Did Not Even Exist	1/15	13%
Did Not Show that Pasteurization Would Have Prevented Outbreak	**15/15**	**100%**

Government officials have perfected their techniques of lying about raw milk to the public. For example, when testing raw milk, they use cultures to promote pathogen multiplication and highly sensitive milk testing techniques that find pathogens in extremely small numbers, levels that would not cause illness (any substance you test will show pathogens if the test is sensitive enough.) Or, they use new rapid testing techniques, such as the PCR test, that err on the side of finding false positives.

When there is an outbreak, they use food questionnaires that leave out likely vectors of disease (such as the local water supply) but always include raw milk. When there is an outbreak, they test raw milk products first, and test samples taken from the home setting rather than unopened cartons from the store shelf. If a person is infected and has handled a raw milk product, the product will test positive for the organism. They then omit testing other foods or raw milk products on the shelf (not handled by the consumer) but report a positive lab result for the opened raw milk product. They can make a case by omitting subjects who got sick but did not drink raw milk; and subjects who drank raw milk but did not get sick. They ignore equally or more likely sources of infection, such as a visit to a farm or petting zoo, tap water, or other foods.

Report of Michigan Fresh Unprocessed Whole Milk Workgroup

They assume that statistical correlation constitutes proof—it is easy to create a statistical association with raw milk using these techniques—and issue inflammatory press releases accusing raw milk, which are not retracted when the dairy is exonerated.

Dr. Beals devised the following analysis on the safety of raw milk. There were an average of 42 government-reported illnesses from raw milk per year for the period 1999-2011.[8] This number includes unconfirmed cases. According to a 2007 CDC survey,[9] there are about 9 million raw milk drinkers in the U.S. (3.04 percent of the population); this number is much higher today. The rate of illness from raw milk can be calculated at .00046%. The actual percentage is probably much lower.

In a population of about 300,000,000, there are about 48,000,000 confirmed cases of foodborne infections per year in the U.S. so the rate of illness from all foods can be calculated at 16 percent.[10]

Thus, you are at least 35,000 times more likely to contract illness from other foods than from raw milk. Plus, drinking raw milk protects you against illness from other foods!

By the way, the largest foodborne illness outbreak in history occurred in the mid-1980s, when almost 200,000 individuals got sick from pasteurized milk in Illinois.

Foodborne illness deaths from dairy products—any dairy product—are extremely rare (although three people died from pasteurized milk in Massachusetts in 2007). Oysters kill something like 15 people per year, and eggs cause 30 illnesses annually. But these are immune from attack—a true double standard.

CDC claims three deaths from raw milk since 2000. One was a cancer patient who didn't drink raw milk although her family did. (Government officials have yet to claim that a raw milk drinker can pass disease to a non-raw milk drinker!) The other two deaths seem to be nonexistent, certainly not reported in the literature.

Report of Michigan Fresh Unprocessed Whole Milk Workgroup

What we do know is that there are about 20 deaths per year from anaphylactic shock to processed milk—probably UHT milk, which is heated to over 280 degrees F.

Why would heat processing make milk so allergenic that it creates anaphylactic shock? No food kills more people this way than heat-processed milk! We find the answer when we look at milk proteins. These are the most complex proteins in nature, three-dimensional and fragile. When heated they become twisted and warped. Not only do they no longer work, but the body sees them as foreign proteins and has to mount an immune response. This explains the various problems—published in the scientific literature—associated with milk consumption, such as juvenile diabetes, asthma, allergies, constipation, frequent ear infections, gastro-intestinal disease and other disorders later in life. Doctors rightly take children off milk—conventional milk—when they suffer from these problems.

The association of milk consumption with disease explains why during a period of rapid population growth, the market for fluid pasteurized milk has declined at 1%-3% per year for the past 30 years. Fewer and fewer consumers can tolerate pasteurized (and ultrapasteurized) milk. The fact is, fewer and fewer people are able to tolerate pasteurized milk; it is one of the top eight allergens and some have violent reactions to it, even causing death.

Meanwhile, consumption of raw milk is rapidly increasing. In several states, there are more dairies producing raw milk than pasteurized. These trends point to the conclusion that eventually more people will be drinking raw milk than pasteurized.

A 2019 paper adds to concerns. Researchers subjected milk to boiling, microwave heating, spray drying, and freeze drying. All four techniques caused oxidative damage to the milk proteins—even freeze-drying! Feeding these damaged milk proteins to rats resulted in learning and memory impairment. Said the researchers,[11] "Processing milk causes the formation of protein oxidation products which impair spatial learning and memory in rats."

Report of Michigan Fresh Unprocessed Whole Milk Workgroup

They concluded, "This means that humans should control milk protein oxidation and improve the processing methods applied to food."[12] What this study indicates is that the only way to "control milk protein oxidation" is to avoid processing altogether and ensure that all milk is sold raw – fresh, unpasteurized whole milk.

Other researchers have looked at the "cytotoxic, genotoxic, mutagenic potential of UHT whole milk."[13] They found ". . . that the long life milk samples caused significant genetic instability to cells of the examined tissue."[14]

The truth is, pasteurization is a rust belt technology—kind of like fighting flies with a sledge hammer. We have beautiful, elegant technologies today that allow us to get clean raw milk to the remotest parts of the country—stainless steel, rapid cooling techniques, on-farm testing, and a national cold chain.

Conventional dairy farmers receive about $1.45 per gallon for milk that costs them $2.00 per gallon to produce. They have no control over this price; they have to take what the dairy company will give them. This is not a sustainable situation, and it explains why the number of licensed dairy operations has declined by more than 55 percent (i.e., from 70,375 in 2003 to 31,657 in 2020).[15] More than 3,000 dairy farms stopped production during 2020 alone— *that's eight per day*. In California, 600 dairy farms were lost in 10 years. The state of Maryland had almost 2,000 dairy farms in 1990; today there are less than 200.[16]

Compulsory pasteurization laws are largely responsible for the decline of American small towns and rural life since pasteurization laws transform what should be a local value-added product that brings prosperity to farmers into a commodity product that enriches the dairy companies and foists bankruptcy on family farms.

Meanwhile, raw dairy farmers get $5 to $25 per gallon with lower costs, and the number of raw dairies is growing! In 1999, our website realmilk.com listed just a couple dozen sources of raw milk in the nation. Today the website lists over

Report of Michigan Fresh Unprocessed Whole Milk Workgroup

3,000! Fewer and fewer folks believe the government anymore. During the intense "bird flu" campaign in California, raw milk sales increased 65 percent.

And raw dairy farms make money! Raw Farm Dairy in California milking 1,800 cows grosses $30 million per year. The Family Cow Dairy in Pennsylvania milks 120 cows and grosses over $2 million per year.[17] Even very small farms can create a decent income for the single mom with a few acres of pasture. If you milk three cows and get 10 gallons per day, sold at $15 per gallon, that's an income of $54,000 per year!

In summary, contrary to the pontifications of government officials, research has shown that there is a very significant difference in the nutritional value of unpasteurized milk versus pasteurized milk. Raw milk is inherently safe; and pasteurization of milk is one of the greatest public health disasters in history.

What's at stake is the health of millions of children worldwide. Raw milk can mean the difference between a healthy productive life and a miserable life.

There's an old saying that truth passes through three phases. First, it is ridiculed. Second, it is violently opposed. Third, it is accepted as self-evident. Thanks to the patience and perception of Dr. Beals and the diligence of the Workgroup, we have entered that third phase. The safety and health benefits of raw milk have become self-evident, and the continued decline of industrial, pasteurized milk is inevitable.

REFERENCES

[1] Sally Fallon Morell. (2024). *The Safety and Health Benefits of Raw Milk,* slide 32 "Decline of Infectious Disease Not Related to Mandatory Pasteurization". (Powerpoint presentation). A Campaign for Real Milk. Accessed 4/10/2025 at https://www.realmilk.com/real-milk-powerpoint/

[2] Ibid, slide 54 "Lowered Nutrient Availability After Pasteurization".

[3] Ibid, slide 36 "Raw Milk and Children - 1926" [from study at a Boston dispensary, *Arch Ped 1926 JUN; 43:380*].

[4] James C. Thomson. (1943). Pasteurised Milk, A National Menace. *The Kingston Chronicle.* Edinburgh, Scotland, p. 5. Accessed 4/10/2025 at https://www.seleneriverpress.com/images/pdfs/Pasteurised_Milk_-_a_National_Menace_-_Scotland_-_JC_THOMSON_1943__Reprint_28C.pdf

[5] Fallon Morell, slide 47 "Raw Milk and Tooth Decay - 1946" [Sprawson quote].

[6] William Campbell Douglas II. (2007). *The Raw Truth About Milk* (formerly, *The Milk Book,* 1984). "Udder Propaganda", Chapter IV. Panama: Rhino Publishing, S.A. Accessed 4/10/2025 at https://ia801203.us.archive.org/11/items/The_Raw_Truth_About_Milk/The_Raw_Truth_About_Milk.pdf

[7] The Weston A. Price Foundation. (2012, March 4). "REBUTTAL TO THE TESTIMONY OF JOHN F. SHEEHAN, BSc (Dy), JD, Director of Plant and Dairy Food Safety, Office of Food Safety, Center for Food Safety and Applied Nutrition, U.S. Food and Drug Administration." p. 11. Accessed 4/10/2025 at https://www.realmilk.com/wp-content/uploads/2000/01/ResponsetoJohnSheehanTestimony.pdf

[8] Ted F. Beals. (2011). Those Pathogens - What You Should Know. (PowerPoint slides). Third International Raw Milk Symposium. slide 22. Accessed 4/11/2025 at https://www.realmilk.com/wp-content/uploads/2012/11/2011_Raw_Milk_Symposium_-_Beals.pdf

[9] Centers for Disease Control and Prevention (CDC). (2007). *Foodborne Diseases Active Surveillance Network (FoodNet) population survey atlas of exposures, 2006-2007.* Atlanta, Georgia: U.S. Department of Health and Human Services, Centers for Disease Control and Prevention, Corporate Authors(s) : National Center for Zoonotic, Vector-Borne, and Enteric Diseases (U.S.). Division of Foodborne, Bacterial, and Mycotic Diseases. Enteric Diseases Epidemiology Branch. p. 14. Accessed 4/11/2025 at https://stacks.cdc.gov/view/cdc/24453

[10] Beals, slide 22.

[11] Li B, Mo L, Yang Y, Zhang S, Xu J, Ge Y, Xu Y, Shi Y, Le G. (2019). Processing milk causes the formation of protein oxidation products which impair spatial learning and memory in rats. *RSC Adv.* 2019 Jul 17;9(39):22161-22175. doi: 10.1039/c9ra03223a. PMID: 35519476; PMCID: PMC9066704. Accessed 4/11/2025 at https://pubs.rsc.org/en/content/articlehtml/2019/ra/c9ra03223a

[12] Ibid.

[13] Brenda de Lima CARVALHO, Ila Monize Sousa SALES and Ana Paula PERON. (2017) Cytotoxic, genotoxic and mutagenic potential of UHT whole milk. *Food Sci. Technol (Campinas).* 2017. Vol. 37(2):275-279. DOI: 10.1590/1678-457x.21916. Accessed 4/11/2025 at https://www.scielo.br/j/cta/a/SJszpWmzbwGtsFR83xjsvRw/?lang=en

[14] Ibid.

[15] Fallon Morell, slide 83 "Industrial Milk Economics".

[16] Ibid, slide 82 "The Wasteland".

[17] Ibid, slide 84 "Raw Milk Economics".

PREFACE

2025 Edition

So, what was the impetus for the Report? It was October 2006 when Michigan State Police and members of the Michigan department of agriculture stopped a truck driven by a farmer and confiscated a large amount of fresh unpasteurized milk on its way to families of a food buyers club—thousands of dollars in dairy and other food products in a sting operation[1] that yielded "450 gallons of raw milk, 29 quarts of fresh cream, 11 quarts of kefir, 4 quarts of buttermilk, 9 quarts of yogurt, and 29 pounds of butter." A criminal referral was made to a Michigan county prosecutor against the farmer alleging violations of the state food code; however, those families had a contractual arrangement to receive their milk and other foods. Nearly 200 club members submitted testimonials[2] about how food from the farmer had benefited their health, including stories of being lactose intolerant[3] and yet having no issues when consuming raw milk. These members and outraged supporters were urging that no charges be brought against the farmer.

The remarkable outcome was ultimately a settlement between the department and the farmer, but more extraordinary was the launching of what turned out to be an unprecedented multi-stakeholder exploration of the benefits and risks of consuming "fresh unprocessed whole milk" (aka, "raw milk"). The six-year process culminated in the legalization of raw milk distribution through herd share arrangements in the State of Michigan by written policy in 2013. The Michigan policy was later tested in a 2016 court case,[4] further illuminating the right of herd share owners to have their portion of raw milk processed into other raw dairy products (e.g., raw cream and raw butter) for their own use; distributing those value-added products back to the owner of the raw milk is also not deemed a "sale" and therefore legal through herd share operations in Michigan.

It's now 2025 and the demand for raw milk throughout the U.S. continues to climb. A 2007 CDC survey[5] revealed that at least 3% of the U.S. population consumed raw milk; undoubtedly, that estimate of 9 million raw milk drinkers has ballooned since then. More states allow not only the distribution of raw milk via herd share arrangements but also allow sales direct to consumers on the farm, through delivery, and--in some states--at other venues such as farmers markets. Many of these states also allow the intrastate distribution of other raw dairy products for human consumption. Even the FDA conceded in 2011[6] that it would not enforce the ban that prohibits the interstate distribution of raw milk for direct human consumption against consumers who cross state lines to obtain raw dairy for their own use. When a federal lawsuit[7] filed by the Farm-to-Consumer Legal Defense Fund was dismissed in 2012, General Counsel Gary Cox triumphantly declared, "Citizens can now purchase raw milk in any state, take it back to their state of residence and consume it without fear of any reprisal from FDA."

Report of Michigan Fresh Unprocessed Whole Milk Workgroup

Why republish a report from 2012 now? The Report was originally printed without copyright so that it could remain accessible in the public domain. Given that both the possession and consumption of any raw dairy product have always been legal throughout the U.S., the Report has been provided to state and federal legislators, regulators and advocates contemplating expanded access in favor of consumer choice and viable market options for dairy farmers. The Report offers the most unbiased in-depth and rigorous examination of the merits and food safety concerns of consuming raw milk and, by extension, holds implications for considering raw dairy products in general, "such as butter, yogurt, cheeses, etc., made from fresh unpasteurized whole milk" which were excluded from the Workgroup's discussions and its recommendations (p. 2). The Workgroup purposely limited its scope to fluid milk in the context of herd share operations with the inherent "rapid trace back" that such a defined pool of consumers offers (p. 142); as such, both the farmer and the consumer share responsibility in maintaining milk quality.

The Report was originally printed by Spring House Press LLC and available for purchase through the Farm-to-Consumer Foundation. With the passing of both Dr. Ted Beals, MD, and his wife Peggy Beals, RN, the Weston A. Price Foundation and the Food Freedom Foundation have taken up the mantle to increase circulation of this vital Report. A Foreword by Sally Fallon Morell and the Afterword by Pete Kennedy contextualize the value of this new edition of the Report which is reproduced here with only minor edits for correcting typos and format adjustments as well as updating online accessibility to cited references where possible.

----

[1] Action Against Raw Milk in Michigan and Indiana. (2006, Oct 27). *Weston A. Price Foundation.* https://www.westonaprice.org/action-against-raw-milk-in-michigan-and-indiana/#gsc.tab=0
[2] Pete Kennedy. (2022, Nov 22). Solari Food Series: Raw Milk Nation. *The Solari Report.* https://home.solari.com/solari-food-series-raw-milk-nation/
[3] Ted Beals. (2008, Mar 29). Pilot Survey of Cow Share Consumer/Owners Lactose Intolerance Section. *RealMilk.com.* https://www.realmilk.com/lactose-intolerance-survey/
[4] Pete Kennedy. (2017, Aug 30). Michigan Raw Dairy – How One Consumer Made an Impact. *RealMilk.com.* https://www.realmilk.com/michigan-raw-dairy-one-consumer-made-impact/
[5] Centers for Disease Control and Prevention (CDC). (2007). *Foodborne Diseases Active Surveillance Network (FoodNet) population survey atlas of exposures, 2006-2007.*
[6,7] Judge Dismisses FDA Raw Milk Lawsuit. (2012, Apr 4). *Farm-to-Consumer Legal Defense Fund.* https://www.farmtoconsumer.org/blog/2012/04/04/judge-dismisses-fda-raw-milk-lawsuit-2/

Report of Michigan Fresh Unprocessed Whole Milk Workgroup

Report
of
Michigan Fresh Unprocessed Whole Milk Workgroup

Presented to Director Jamie Clover Adams
Michigan Department of Agriculture and Rural Development

December 11, 2012

Michigan Fresh Unprocessed Whole Milk Workgroup

RECOMMENDATIONS

Approved December 11, 2012

General considerations of the Fresh Unprocessed Whole Milk Workgroup's recommendations:

- During the Workgroup's deliberations, herd share programs were considered to include only Fresh Unprocessed Whole (FUW) milk intended for human consumption.
- Products such as butter, yogurt, cheeses, etc., made from fresh unprocessed milk were not included in the workgroup's discussions and are not included in these recommendations.
- The Workgroup recommends that herd share programs not be regulated and that legislation is not needed to implement these recommendations.
- State and local health agencies should maintain their current ability to investigate food and health issues.
- There is a need for further education on herd shares and FUW milk.
- Representatives from the Workgroup would remain available as a resource.
- The herd share farmers and shareholders should be made aware of the FUW milk Workgroup's recommendations and report.

The Workgroup recommends that herd share operations include the following elements:

- There must be a signed and dated written contract between a single herd share farmer and shareholder.
- There must be a workable means of communication between the farmer and all of the households receiving milk.
- Milk should be from a single farm and not mixed with another farm's milk.

The Workgroup recommends the following scope of herd share arrangements:

- FUW milk is not for sale or resale.
- Shareholders should be encouraged to periodically pick up the FUW milk from the farm.

Report of Michigan Fresh Unprocessed Whole Milk Workgroup

- The herd share farmer should provide educational material about the farm, including farm operations, benefits, risks, and responsibilities, all of which should be in the contract.
- FUW milk cannot be distributed from a licensed food establishment.
- Advertising of herd shares is not regulated.

Why the Workgroup is comfortable with these recommendations:

- There is a defined consumer pool.
- Rapid trace back is possible.
- The farmer and shareholder are both responsible for maintaining the quality of the milk.
- The Workgroup wants the shareholder to be knowledgeable about the operation of the herd share.
- The Michigan Fresh Unprocessed Whole Milk Workgroup report will be available to the farmers and shareholders.

Recommended Next Steps:

- Meet with the MDARD Director to discuss the FUW milk Workgroup recommendations and next steps.
- Request that the Food and Dairy Division develop a guidance document for its staff, built on these recommendations. This guidance document will be shared with the Michigan FUW milk stakeholders.
- The Michigan Fresh Unprocessed Whole Milk Workgroup requests that representatives of the Workgroup be included in any discussion on changes to MDARD's stance regarding FUW milk.

About the Michigan Fresh Unprocessed Whole Milk Workgroup

Purpose

The Workgroup is addressing the question: ***"Where do we want to be in 3 to 5 years in terms of access to fresh unprocessed whole milk?"***

Goal

The group desires clear direction, with clear public policy, regarding access to fresh unprocessed whole milk and, if needed, adjust the law accordingly.

Background

In Michigan in October 2006, the question of access to raw milk came to a head when the Michigan Department of Agriculture (now known as the Michigan Department of Agriculture and Rural Development: MDARD) initiated an investigation and legal action against a food cooperative for, among other things, the distribution of unpasteurized milk and milk products. As a result, Michigan Food and Farming Systems (MIFFS) and Michigan State University (MSU) met with MDARD leadership to discuss the action and how to address a desire among some Michigan consumers for access to raw milk while, at the same time, minimizing health risks.

It was decided that a Workgroup would be formed, and the first meeting was held in January 2007. Workgroup members represent an array of perspectives, relative to the issue at hand and the group's purpose: consumers who seek to ensure access to raw milk; producers who want to provide a healthy source of raw milk; a Grade "A" milk industry representative and food safety regulators who are looking to balance access and choice issues, while protecting the food supply.

MIFFS and MSU served as facilitators and resource providers to guide the dialog and deliberations of the Workgroup.

The group agreed to use the term Fresh Unprocessed Whole Milk to describe the product intended for direct human consumption, since "raw milk" is used to describe milk intended for pasteurization. The group agreed to address the question: "Where do we want to be in 3 to 5 years on access to fresh unprocessed whole milk?"

The Michigan Fresh Unprocessed Whole Milk Workgroup met to identify issues and questions regarding access to this milk. The Workgroup reached consensus on the goal: **"The group desires clear direction with clear**

Report of Michigan Fresh Unprocessed Whole Milk Workgroup

public policy regarding access to fresh unprocessed whole milk and, if needed, adjust the law accordingly." The group decided to reach this goal using a question-and-answer format. Over 60 questions covering 10 topic areas were initially identified by the Workgroup. Since early 2007, the group has met almost monthly in face-to-face, usually three-hour sessions to discuss the questions, share resources and expertise, and develop answers to the questions. An additional five-hour meeting was held with herd share farmers to solicit their views, needs, and ideas. The group invited guest speakers to share information and expertise which aided the development of answers to the questions. The Michigan Fresh Unprocessed Whole Milk Workgroup's answers to the questions were developed after thorough discussion, deliberation, and consensus among the group's members. As time went on, some of the topics and questions originally developed were removed from the Workgroup's consideration because they were no longer relevant to the goal.

By agreement, the group's discussions have been kept confidential. However, as each topic was completed, the consensus summary was posted on a website made available by MIFFS. The Workgroup's discussions and resulting recommendations are focused on the state of Michigan. The questions, answers, recommendations, and additional reference information are included in this report.

Since 2007, some members of the Workgroup have retired while other members have joined it. Over this time, Workgroup members have celebrated milestone birthdays, wedding anniversaries, graduations, and births of children and grandchildren. The Workgroup members have especially enjoyed the opportunity to get to know each other and understand differing perspectives on the subject of consumer access to fresh unprocessed whole milk.

Report of Michigan Fresh Unprocessed Whole Milk Workgroup

Michigan Fresh Unprocessed Whole Milk Workgroup Members

Elaine Brown, Executive Director, Michigan Food & Farming Systems, January 2007-Dec 2011 (Moderator)

Ted Beals, MD, Retired pathologist, faculty U of Mich. Med. School; Director, Farm-to-Consumer Foundation; and MI Fresh Milk Council, January 2007-present

Peggy Beals, RN, Teacher, lecturer, and author: Traditional Food Preparation and Food Safety; Leader, South Central Michigan Chapter, Weston A. Price Foundation; Nonpaid Administrator and member, MI Fresh Milk Council; and Director, Farm-to-Consumer Foundation, January 2007-present

Susan Esser, Food and Dairy Division Deputy Director, Michigan Department of Agriculture and Rural Development, January 2007-present

Frank Fear, Sr., PhD, Associate Dean, MSU College of Agriculture and Natural Resources and Kettering Project Principal, January 2007-Dec 2011

Katherine Fedder, Director, Food and Dairy Division, Michigan Department of Agriculture, January 2007-December 2010

Jesse and Betsy Meerman, Cow Share Dairy Farmers, March 2011-present

Jennifer Nord, Environmental Sanitarian, University of Michigan, September 2011- present

John Partridge, PhD, Michigan State University, Department of Food Science and Human Nutrition, May 2011-present

Rosanne Ponkowski, Executive Director, Healthy Traditions Network, Metro Detroit Chapter, Weston A. Price Foundation and Member of MI Fresh Milk Council, January 2007-present

Joe Scrimger, Principle, Bio-Systems; Life Time Foods; Scrimger Farm and Member MI Fresh Milk Council; Member of Healthy Traditions Network; and Chair of Michigan Thumb Organics (MTO), January 2007-present

Gary Trimner, Director of Member Services, Michigan Milk Producers Association, January 2007-December 2011

John and Patti Warnke, Cow Share Dairy Farmers and Members MI Fresh Milk Council, January 2007-June 2011

Invited Subject Matter Experts

George Bird, PhD, Professor, Michigan State University, Department of Entomology

Edwin Blosser, Owner, Midwest Bio-Systems

Tilak Dhiman, PhD, Animal Nutrition, Environmental Health and Natural Foods

Angela Renee Katafiasz, DVM, private veterinary practitioner

Paul Bartlett, MPH, DVM, PhD, Michigan State University, Department of Large Animal Clinical Science, College of Veterinary Medicine

Mark McAfee, California Certified Raw Milk Organic Dairy Farmer

Greg Miller, PhD, Vice-President, National Dairy Council

Sally Fallon Morell, President and Treasurer, Weston A. Price Foundation

Elliot Ryser, PhD, Michigan State University, Department of Food Science and Human Nutrition

Melinda Wilkins, PhD, Director, Communicable Disease Division, Michigan Department of Community Health

Warnke Family, Warnke's Emerald Acres Farm

Discussion Summaries

Michigan Fresh Unprocessed Whole Milk Workgroup

Topic 1

History
of
Fresh Unprocessed
Whole Milk

1. Historically, why is milk an important component of our diet?

2. What is the history of milk regulation?

3. Why is milk one of the most regulated foods in the U.S.?

4. Is there something uniquely hazardous about milk?

5. Initially, what were the conditions that prompted pasteurization for milk – have those conditions and knowledge/understanding changed today?

Summary
Approved June 8, 2009

Topic 1 – History of Fresh Unprocessed Milk

1. Historically, why is milk an important component of our diet?

"It has been said truly that milk is the only material in the whole range of animal matter that is designed and prepared by nature expressly as food." (From the preface to the 6th Annual Meeting of the American Association of Medical Milk Commissions, 1916)

As far back as we have recorded evidence, milk and milk products have been a mainstay of infant, child, and adult diets. Earliest records document the domestication of animals as a source of fluid milk and other dairy products, and religious texts contain many references to milk.

Historians have repeatedly cited ways in which the consumption of milk was a competitive advantage for people. It was a rich source of nutrients and water. Domesticated lactating animals accompanied migrating people and moved with armies as they marched across great distances. Many of the early settlers to this country brought dairy animals with them to provide milk during their transatlantic crossings and in their new communities. Traditionally, nearly all milk was obtained directly from the animal, was consumed fresh, and was not refrigerated.

Milk-producing animals were prevalent throughout the world and intentionally bred to produce more milk than was needed for human consumption for newborns. Fresh milk proved palatable and nutritionally beneficial. It was also cultured into many foods, such as yogurt and kefir (a fermented milk drink) and preserved as butter, ghee (butterfat separated from milk), and a variety of cheeses. This practice increased the nutrient content and portability of these products and extended their storage life, which helped sustain people during harsh times and when animals weren't producing milk. Milk-producing animals were considered – and still are – a sign of personal wealth and security. In some cultures, the cow is considered sacred.

Historically, milk consumption was common and unregulated. Recorded history does not show that milk caused widespread disease. Traditional diets, developed over generations, remain if they are beneficial and do not have adverse consequences.

2.   What is the history of milk regulation?

In the U.S., milk and milk products were not regulated until the 20th century. Milk-producing animals were prevalent and well integrated into the community, family life and local commerce.

Then several things happened:
- There was a huge increase in the population of metropolitan areas, resulting from the influx of immigrants and people moving to urban areas for work.

- New dairies were located near these rapidly growing urban centers to meet the demand of milk to these huge concentrations of people. The industrial model was seen by these urban dairies as a way to maximize profits by efficiencies of scale and the use of locally-available, cheap, alternative feed.

- Dairies developed extensive distribution systems to reach consumers. Some milk production facilities located in cities still obtained milk from rural dairies, requiring transportation of farm milk over considerable distances. Farmers left cans of milk on platforms beside railroad tracks, and trains would stop and pick the cans up along the way. This is the origin of the term "milk run" – a train that made repeated stops to pick up cans of milk. This expanded movement of milk resulted in longer times between milking and public consumption. None of this milk was refrigerated.

- As the demand for milk in these urban areas increased, a few dairies exploited the situation to increase profits. Examples included adding water to augment volume, using whiteners to hide discoloration, and adding disinfectants to camouflage spoilage.

During this same period, a number of diseases developed into serious public health problems due to overcrowding, inadequate means to dispose of human waste, and rudimentary water and sewage treatment. Scientists began to understand that microorganisms were often the cause of these illnesses.

Federal food safety regulation began when farmers called for a national approach to meat processing in order to be able to compete on the foreign market, resulting in the Meat Inspection Act of 1891. At the time, domestic and European markets were being threatened by growing public concern over diseases such as trichinosis from pork.

The public became outraged when journalists reported the unsanitary conditions in "swill dairies" (so named because they were located near distilleries to take advantage of huge amounts of waste material—known as swill—left over from fermenting grains). The swill was used as a substitute for pasture/forage feeding.

Report of Michigan Fresh Unprocessed Whole Milk Workgroup

Newspapers showed pictures of milk transporters adding water to milk cans and other questionable practices to increase profits (now categorized as adulteration and mislabeling). Groups of physicians made the connection between unsanitary conditions at dairies and children developing diarrhea when consuming bottled milk.

In 1892 a New York physician, Dr. Henry Coit, introduced a system for designating milk from inspected dairy farms as "Certified Milk". As a strong proponent of pasteurization, Nathan Straus contributed some of his personal wealth to building milk pasteurization plants and distribution centers in large cities as a way of providing subsidized "pure" milk to the poor, particularly for newborns of mothers who were not able to breast feed. Soon 20 large cities had distribution centers, half required pasteurization, all used only Certified Milk. There was vigorous public and scientific debate about the "milk problem". Some milk processors saw the advantages of pasteurization (e.g., extended time to transport milk, reduced spoilage, and marketing their milk as germ-free), but the physician groups were concerned that pasteurization destroyed medical benefits of the milk. Physicians, veterinarians and health officials argued that the solution to the unsanitary conditions and public health issues was to encourage dairies to clean up in order to meet the Medical Milk Commissions' certification standards. This was a prolonged and contentious debate.

During the first decade of the 20th century, there was an increase in the number of local governments that adopted strict sanitation standards. Many of the Medical Milk Commissions included a requirement for testing cows for tuberculosis, using a new test. In Chicago, this resulted in municipal regulations requiring that milk from cows not tested for tuberculosis be pasteurized. Most of the local regulations and laws for sanitation standards were later expanded by, initially, recommending and then requiring pasteurization.

In 1906, the Federal Food and Drug Act was passed. Most large cities had pasteurization requirements by 1917. In 1924, the U.S. Public Health Service developed a model regulation known as the Standard Milk Ordinance for voluntary adoption by state and local agencies. This model regulation is now known as the Grade "A" Pasteurized Milk Ordinance (PMO) and has been adopted by nearly every state. In 1948, Michigan became the first state to require pasteurization of all sold milk. There were still Medical Milk Commissions in the 1970s and 1980s.

3. Why is milk one of the most regulated foods in the U.S.?

Food regulation in the United States has a complex history which started with the discovery of microorganisms that were linked to communicable diseases. There was a common school of thought during the late 19th and early 20th century that, by eradicating germs, we could eliminate disease. This idea was promoted by a variety of advocacy groups. Due to its widespread consumption, milk was one of the earliest foods to stimulate debate related to food safety. Historically, milk regulations were linked to the "war on germs". In addition, early milk regulations targeted areas such as the adulteration of milk and dairy products, the health of milk-producing animals, and the health of people involved in handling milk and dairy products.

In 1924, the U.S. Public Health Service developed a model regulation known as the Standard Milk Ordinance for voluntary adoption by state and local agencies. With the addition of the pasteurization step in the processing of milk, a whole new set of regulations were needed to maintain the effectiveness of the pasteurization process. As imitation dairy products were made commercially available, the general public as well as manufacturers began demanding controls covering mislabeling. Various state and local governments developed their own regulations governing milk and dairy products, sometimes with the intent of protecting their local dairies from competing dairies in others cities or states. Following World War II, the problem of regulatory barriers to the free flow of milk between markets increased, leading to the formation of the National Conference on Interstate Milk Shipments (NCIMS) in 1950.

The NCIMS provides cooperative input for the states, the dairy industry, and the Food and Drug Administration regarding milk regulation. All proposed changes to the PMO filter through the committee structure of the NCIMS and are voted on by representatives of state regulatory agencies. The NCIMS meets every two years and, typically, over 100 proposals for changes to the PMO and other NCIMS documents are reviewed. These proposals are submitted by states, industry and the FDA. The NCIMS promotes regulatory uniformity across the United States, allowing milk regulatory issues to be thoroughly discussed by stakeholders and alleviating the need for individual states to enact their own dairy laws. In 2004, the Institute of Health in their report, "Scientific Criteria to Ensure Safe Food", made a point about the historical background of food regulation: "The need for such standards in the food industry goes to the heart of regulatory theory, which recognizes the necessity for the government to establish standards as a counterbalance to private economic incentives." The PMO, along with the NCIMS program, are recognized by the FDA as a state and federal cooperative program providing milk regulatory oversight for the entire U.S.

The PMO includes both technology-based and performance-based standards. For example, the construction standards for the floors, walls and ceilings of a dairy

---

Report of Michigan Fresh Unprocessed Whole Milk Workgroup

plant have been included in the PMO and have changed very little over the past 55 years. Performance standards such as cooling temperatures, bacteria and coliform counts have also been included in the PMO over the years. The NCIMS process allows for the adoption of new systems and technology. For example, in 2003, a voluntary Hazard Analysis Critical Control Point Program for dairy plants was adopted and, more recently, standards for automatic (robotic) milking systems have been added to the PMO. The document has evolved into a complex and comprehensive set of regulations.

The PMO requirements are limited to Grade "A" milk and milk products intended for shipment across state lines. However, states have the authority to regulate milk and milk products that move within their borders. Some states adopt, and may even expand, the PMO requirements as state law to cover intrastate sales. Other dairy products, such as ice cream and cheese, are regulated by individual states.

4. Is there something uniquely hazardous about milk?

Milk is not inherently hazardous. Fresh milk from the mammary glands is one of the most nutritious and complete foods available to humans. Although milk contains water and many other nutrients to sustain growth of bacteria—whether beneficial or pathogenic—many other foods have similar characteristics that can readily support the growth of disease-producing bacteria: fresh and processed meat, seafood, and foods consumed fresh, such as produce, coconut milk, and fruit juices. To enhance safe products, animal-based products require good handling practices. Milk is a liquid that is harvested from animals at a body temperature conducive to bacterial contamination from the environment. No food, including milk, is completely safe.

5. Initially, what were the conditions that prompted pasteurization for milk – have those conditions and knowledge/understanding changed today?

At the turn of the 20th century, much of the public concern around disease and dissatisfaction with milk was caused by the swill dairies in large urban areas and the human illness caused by milk that was contaminated by sick cows, sick humans, unsanitary handling, and adulteration. Doctors in orphanages noticed that children were becoming ill from drinking milk. Filthy dairy operations, with both sick animals and sick or unclean workers, led to heavily soiled and contaminated milk. The initial milk commission criteria for certification focused primarily on these conditions. Public outrage, certification criteria, and subsequent adoption of these standards into milk regulations resulted in considerable improvement in the sanitation and cleanliness of dairies.

Report of Michigan Fresh Unprocessed Whole Milk Workgroup

Much of the public concern about disease and dissatisfaction with milk was caused by long-distance transportation, mostly unrefrigerated (trains to bottling plants and bottled milk to retail outlets or homes). Milk spoiled, but it's important to clarify that spoiled milk is not hazardous—it is simply unmarketable. The heightened awareness of the importance of refrigeration and manufacturer's testing protocols has improved considerably in recent years. "Pasteurization", which was at that time some sort of heat treatment, helped the manufacturers by enabling more time to transport, process, and store milk by killing spoilage organisms.

Other advocates for pasteurization were coming forward from individuals concerned with infant mortality, such as Nathan Strauss. Pasteurization was seen by some public health officials as a quick, cost-effective way to eliminate pathogens in milk.

Epidemics publicly perceived to be associated with drinking milk at that time, including brucellosis (known as Bangs or undulant fever), diphtheria, typhoid, and tuberculosis, spread mostly in urban areas that lacked sanitation. All of these serious diseases are now under control; diphtheria and typhoid by treatment of people who were spreading the disease and improved sanitation requirements for food and water. Brucellosis and bovine tuberculosis were controlled by a massive program of testing and depopulation of cattle. These are all public health successes resulting from federally mandated disease eradication policies.

Conditions have changed considerably since the early 20th century in terms of sanitation and public health. Our knowledge of what it takes to maintain the quality and safety of milk has grown, including our understanding of good herd management, disease-causing and healthy bacteria, our ability to test for pathogens, the capacity to rapidly chill milk and give attention to constant refrigeration, the use of stainless steel, improved design of processing equipment, and improved cleaning techniques. Regulations at the state and federal level have and continue to improve milk quality and safety, as do dairy farmers and milk processors.

Report of Michigan Fresh Unprocessed Whole Milk Workgroup

References

Untold Story of Milk, Ron Schmid. New Trends Publishing, 2003.

Nature's Perfect Food: How Milk became America's Drink, E. Melanie Dupuis, NYU press, 2002.

Committee on the Review of the Use of Scientific Criteria and Performance Standards for Safe Food. *Scientific Criteria to Ensure Safe Food.* Chapter 1, "Historical Perspective on the Use of Food Safety Criteria and Performance Standards"; Institute of Medicine Research Council. The National Academies Press, 2003. Cited url: http://books.nap.edu/openbook.php?record id=10690&page=13 [Redirected to: https://nap.nationalacademies.org/read/10690/chapter/3]

Henry I. Coit and the Certified Milk Movement in the Development of Modern Pediatrics, Manfred J. Waserman. ProQuest Information and Learning Co. Johns Hopkins University Press, 2003. Bull Hist Med.; 46 (4):359-90 1972. Cited url: http://www.ncbi.nlm.nih.gov/pubmed/4562983 [Redirected to: https://pubmed.ncbi.nlm.nih.gov/4562983/]

Sixth Annual Meeting of the American Association of Medical Milk Commissions, 1912. https://books.google.com/books?id=cqYDAAAAYAAJ&dq=+henry+coit+certified+milk+movement&source=gbssummarys&cad=O

Food and Drug Administration Milestones in U.S. Food and Drug Law History, 2005. Cited url: http://www.fda.gov/opacom/backgrounders/miles.html [Revised url: https://www.fda.gov/about-fda/fda-history/milestones-us-food-and-drug-law]

History and Accomplishments of the National Conference on Interstate Milk Shipments, 2001 Edition, National Conference on Interstate Milk Shipments, 123 Buena Vista Drive, Frankfort, KY 40601. Cited url: http://www.ncims.org [Revision, 2009 ed.: https://ncims.org/wp-content/uploads/2018/10/History-and-Accomplishments-of-the-NCIMS-through-2009.pdf]

Pure Milk is Better Than Purified Milk, Alan Czaplicki, Social Science History, 31:3 Fall 2007, pages 411-433.

John Partridge, PhD, Michigan State University, Department of Food Science and Human Nutrition. Workgroup interview on March 11, 2008.

Topic 2

Benefits
and
Values

1. What is the nutritional value of milk?

2. Going beyond the Nutrition Facts Label –
   What other nutritional values should we
   be considering?

3. What are the additional benefits of milk
   fresh from the cow?

4. What is the impact of pasteurization on
   the value of FUW milk?

5. What is the impact of homogenization on
   the value of FUW milk?

6. Assuming that all milk is not the same,
   what do production and management
   practices have to do with FUW milk's
   nutritional value, pathogens, color, taste,
   etc.?

7. What is the impact of consumer
   preferences on production and
   management practices of FUW milk?

Summary

Approved April 20, 2010

Topic 2 – Benefits and Values

1. What is the nutritional value of milk?

Milk is a complete food. It serves as the sole nourishment and fluid for newborns during a most critical stage of their development. It is an important part of most children's diet, with dairy products providing calcium and many other nutrients needed for a growing child.

For adults, milk is a readily available source of numerous essential nutrients including high-quality, low-cost protein, a minimum of carbohydrate and an appropriate balance of fatty acids. Milk is considered an excellent source of calcium, phosphorous, vitamins B-2 and D-3, and a good source of fat, carbohydrate, protein, vitamin C, and the B vitamin, folate.

The taste of milk is generally enjoyable, and this pleasure enhances its digestibility.

Nutritional Facts labels list the quantities of certain nutrients in food. The amount of a nutrient is listed as a measured weight, such as in grams (g), milligrams (mg), or International Units (IU). The other way of indicating proportions is to list a compound using a complicated formula, based on an estimated intake of a 2,000 or 2,500 calorie diet, and is indicated as a Percent Daily Value number (%DV). The energy we derive from food is measured in calories and is listed for fat, carbohydrates, and protein on the label. The calorie number is based on the serving size, listed at the top of the label, multiplied by the

Nutrition Facts

Serving Size 8fl oz (240mL)
Servings Per Container 8

Amount Per Serving

Calories 150	Calories from Fat 70

	% Daily Value*
Total Fat 8g	**12%**
Saturated Fat 5g	**25%**
Trans Fat 0g	
Cholesterol 35mg	**11%**
Sodium 120mg	**5%**
Potassium 390mg	**11%**
Total Carbohydrates 12g	**4%**
Dietary Fibre 0g	**0%**
Sugars 11g	
Protein 8g	

Vitamin A 6%	•	Vitamin C 4%
Calcium 30%	•	Iron 0%
Vitamin D 25%		

* Percent Daily Values are based on a 2,000 calorie diet. Your daily values may be higher or lower depending on your calorie needs:

		Calories	2,000	2,500
Total Fat	Less than		65g	60g
Sat Fat	Less than		20g	25g
Cholesterol	Less than		300mg	300mg
Sodium	Less than		2,400mg	2,400mg
Potassium			3,500mg	3,500mg
Total Carbohydrate			300g	375g
Dietary Fiber			25g	30g

INGREDIENTS: ORGANIC MILK, AND VITAMIN D3

CONTAINS: MILK

calories per gram:

Fat – 9 calories/gram
Carbohydrate – 4 calories/gram, and
Protein – 4 calories/gram

(Tables of Nutritional Facts x 3)

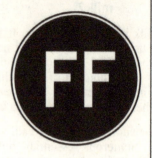

Nutrition Facts
Serving Size 8fl oz (240mL)
Servings Per Container 4

Amount Per Serving	
Calories 90	Calories from Fat 0
	% Daily Value*
Total Fat 0g	0%
Saturated Fat 0g	0%
Trans Fat 0g	
Cholesterol 5mg	1%
Sodium 130mg	5%
Potassium 410mg	12%
Total Carbohydrates 13g	4%
Dietary Fibre 0g	0%
Sugars 12g	
Protein 8g	17%

Vitamin A 10% • Vitamin C 4%
Calcium 30% • Iron 0%
Vitamin D 25%

* Percent Daily Values are based on a 2,000 calorie diet. Your daily values may be higher or lower depending on your calorie needs:

	Calories	2,000	2,500
Total Fat	Less than	65g	60g
Sat Fat	Less than	20g	25g
Cholesterol	Less than	300mg	300mg
Sodium	Less than	2,400mg	2,400mg
Potassium		3,500mg	3,500mg
Total Carbohydrate		300g	375g
Dietary Fiber		25g	30g
Protein		50g	65g

Calories per gram
Fat 9 - Carbohydrate 4 - Protein 4

Fat Free Milk

Vitamin A & D
Grade A
Pasteurized
Homogenized

INGREDIENTS:
FAT FREE MILK, VITAMIN A PALMITATE, VITAMIN D3

KEEP REFRIGERATED

Fat Free Milk

Vitamin A & D

Grade A

1 QUART (946mL)

Report of Michigan Fresh Unprocessed Whole Milk Workgroup

Nutrition Facts	
Serving Size 8fl oz (240mL)	
Servings Per Container 4	

Amount Per Serving	
Calories 130	Calories from Fat 45
	% Daily Value*
Total Fat 5g	8%
Saturated Fat 3g	15%
Trans Fat 3g	
Cholesterol 20mg	7%
Sodium 130mg	5%
Potassium 400mg	11%
Total Carbohydrates 12g	4%
Dietary Fibre 0g	0%
Sugars 12g	
Protein 8g	17%

Vitamin A 10%	•	Vitamin C 4%
Calcium 30%	•	Iron 0%
Vitamin D 25%		

* Percent Daily Values are based on a 2,000 calorie diet. Your daily values may be higher or lower depending on your calorie needs:

	Calories	2,000	2,500
Total Fat	Less than	65g	60g
Sat Fat	Less than	20g	25g
Cholesterol	Less than	300mg	300mg
Sodium	Less than	2,400mg	2,400mg
Potassium		3,500mg	3,500mg
Total Carbohydrate		300g	305g
Dietary Fiber		25g	30g
Protein		50g	65g

Calories per gram
Fat 9 - Carbohydrate 4 - Protein 4

2% Reduced Fat Milk
37% LESS FAT THAN REGULAR MILK

Vitamin A & D
2% Milkfat
Grade A
Pasteurized
Homogenized

Fat reduced from 8g to 5g per serving.

INGREDIENTS:
REDUCED FAT MILK,
VITAMIN A, PALMITATE,
VITAMIN D3

KEEP REFRIGERATED

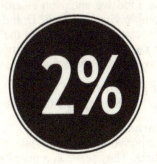

2% Reduced Fat Milk

Vitamin A & D
2% Milkfat

Grade A

1 QUART (946mL)

Nutritional Components Listed on Nutrition Facts Label

Fats
Fats consist of a large group of compounds that are made up of fatty acids (saturated and unsaturated). Fats are generally soluble in organic solvents and largely insoluble in water. Fats support and cushion organs and protect nerves. Nutritionally, fats are the source of essential fatty acids. In nutritional terms, an

Report of Michigan Fresh Unprocessed Whole Milk Workgroup

essential substance is one that cannot be produced by the body so it must come from the food we eat. Non-essential substances can be synthesized internally. The fat-soluble vitamins A, E, D and K, can only be digested, absorbed and transported in association with fats, and the body can store these vitamins in fatty tissue. Milk fat in dairy products is the carrier of these fat-soluble vitamins, as well as important flavor and aroma substances.

The fat content of commercial milk is typically standardized at: ½%, 1%, 2%, or 3.25%. See representative labels on previous page.

Carbohydrates
Carbohydrates are organic compounds that include sugars, starches, cellulose, and gums. They serve as a major energy source. The main carbohydrate in milk is sugar lactose.

Protein
Proteins are large organic compounds composed of amino acid chains. Proteins are utilized in every physiological process within the body. Milk is a complete protein – it contains all eight essential amino acids as well as some non-essential ones.

The most plentiful protein in milk is casein. Casein proteins are unique to milk and milk products; they are not found in any other foods.

Vitamins and Minerals
Vitamins are organic substances required for many physiological processes. Milk contains fat-soluble vitamins A, D, E, and K. Vitamins A and D work as a team, so both must be available in the proper proportion and at the same time to be assimilated. Milk is also an important source of several water-soluble vitamins: B-1 (thiamine), B-2 (riboflavin), B-3 (niacin), B-6 (pyridoxine), B-12 (cobalamin), and pantothenic acid.

All 22 minerals considered to be essential to the human diet are present in milk. Milk supplies these minerals in the correct proportions. Calcium, magnesium, and potassium are needed together for healthy bones. They also serve to regulate nerve connectivity and muscle and nerve contractions.

Appropriate balances of these minerals prevent misfiring and cramping of muscles, including the muscles of the heart. Sodium, potassium, and chloride serve to maintain the osmotic equilibrium of milk with blood.

There is very little difference in the calcium content of reduced-fat dairy products compared to those made with whole milk.

Report of Michigan Fresh Unprocessed Whole Milk Workgroup

Nutrition Facts

Serving Size 1 cup (240mL)
Servings Per Container 4

Amount Per Serving

Calories 150	Calories from Fat 70
	% Daily Value*
Total Fat 8g	12%
Saturated Fat 5g	25%
Trans Fat 0g	
Cholesterol 35mg	11%
Sodium 120mg	5%
Potassium 380mg	11%
Total Carbohydrates 12g	4%
Dietary Fibre 0g	0%
Sugars 11g	
Protein 8g	16%

Vitamin A 6%	•	Vitamin C 4%
Calcium 30%	•	Iron 0%
Vitamin D 25%		

*Percent Daily Values are based on a 2,000 calorie diet. Your daily values may be higher or lower depending on your calorie needs:

	Calories	2,000	2,500
Total Fat	Less than	65g	60g
Sat Fat	Less than	20g	25g
Cholesterol	Less than	300mg	300mg
Sodium	Less than	2,400mg	2,400mg
Potassium		3,500mg	3,500mg
Total Carbohydrate		300g	375g
Dietary Fiber		25g	30g
Protein		50g	65g

Calories per gram
Fat 9 - Carbohydrate 4 - Protein 4

Vitamin D Milk

Grade A
Pasteurized
Homogenized
3.25% Milkfat

INGREDIENTS:
MILK, VITAMIN D3

KEEP REFRIGERATED

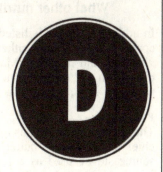

Vitamin D Milk

Grade A

1 QUART (946mL)

Report of Michigan Fresh Unprocessed Whole Milk Workgroup

2. Going beyond the Nutrition Facts label – What other nutritional values should we be considering?

In addition to what is listed on conventional nutrition labels, we find that milk is complex and contains other required, interdependent elements such as enzymes, vitamins, and minerals. Many of these elements are absorbed intact and function directly in our metabolism. Others serve to foster the bioavailability of the basic nutrients – fats, carbohydrates, and proteins – in the milk.

Fats
The fat in whole milk has many benefits. Butterfat is the natural fat of milk. It is the chief component of butter. Historically, it is one of the first fats from animal sources to be used as a food. Butterfat is good for the bones and enhances the immune system. It is directly absorbed, thus giving quick energy instead of being laid down as body fat for future utilization. In addition, fat in the diet gives an increased satiety value by slowing absorption of the food eaten. The slow digestion of fat provides gradual energy and allows the body to absorb needed nutrients along with the fat. The good satiety of whole milk may contribute to eating appropriate amounts of food, i.e., not overeating.

Each butterfat globule is surrounded by a membrane consisting of phospholipids and proteins. These emulsifiers keep the individual globules of butterfat from joining together into clumps, as well as protecting the globules from the fat-digesting activity of enzymes found in the fluid portion of milk.

In addition to the conventionally listed fats, Omega 3 and Omega 6 fatty acids also occur in whole milk.

The scientific community is looking closely at Conjugated Linoleic Acid (CLA). CLA is a unique fatty acid that is formed in the rumen, the first chamber of the cow and sheep's digestive system that allows them, by bacterial action, to utilize fresh grass as their primary food. The amount of CLA in milk depends on the breed of the animal, its feed and environment, and the season. Researchers are excited by the possibility of CLA being effective in cancer prevention, particularly in breast and prostate cancer. Research is suggestive that CLA may strengthen the immune system, and it may also have properties that tend to normalize body fat deposition.

The fat in whole milk contributes 48%-50% of the calories, and most of the flavor, of milk.

"There is no evidence that moderate intake of milk fat gives increased risk of diseases." - Anna Haug, et al "Bovine milk in human nutrition - a review."

Carbohydrates
Milk has a glycemic index number of 30. Foods with a number below 55 are considered "low" and are therefore good choices for a sugar-restricted diet, such as

---

Report of Michigan Fresh Unprocessed Whole Milk Workgroup

diabetes. Another plus is that 8 ounces of milk contains 12 grams of sugar, a commonly recommended target amount for a snack.

Protein

"The protein in milk has a quality higher than many other foods, but the quantity of milk protein is low due to high water content. Milk protein contains all the essential amino acids required by the body for optimum growth; for this reason, more of the protein can be used for protein anabolism, so there's less chance the protein in milk will be converted to fat and stored." - American Dairy Science Association, 1999.

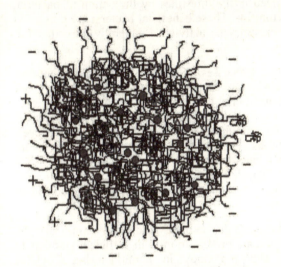

The hairy casein micelle model, referred to as the Holt Hairy Model, where a spherical, tangled web and open structure of polypeptide chains cross-link by calcium phosphate nanocluster (colloidal calcium phosphate) in the core, provides rise to an external region of lower segment density known as the hairy layer. The embedded gray circles represent the calcium phosphate nanoclusters.

The protein casein represents about 80% of milk protein. Caseins are a large group of related proteins that are bound together with calcium phosphate into aggregates known as micelles (pronounced MY cells). Micelles contain a mixture of the various caseins, as well as the calcium, magnesium, and inorganic phosphorus needed to build bone, muscle, and tissue. The structure and composition of micelles make the casein proteins and the salts of the minerals calcium (Ca), magnesium (Mg) and inorganic Phosphorus (P) more bioavailable. They also form a curd (dabber) in the stomach for slower, more efficient digestion.

There are dozens of other proteins in milk that are more water-soluble than caseins. Because these other proteins remain suspended in the whey left behind when the caseins coagulate into curds, as in cheese-making, they are collectively known as whey proteins. Whey protein is absorbed rapidly, resulting in high concentrations of amino acids in the blood stream for ready energy and muscle strength. Excess calories from carbohydrates and protein, not just fat, are made into fat by the liver and adipose tissue. By the same token, high quality protein, appropriate amounts of carbohydrates and good fat, all contribute to the feeling of satisfaction after a meal.

Other Nutrients

Enzymes act as catalysts, contributing to nutrient availability (bioavailability). In whole or complete foods such as milk, the enzymes that are needed to digest a compound usually occur along with the compound. For example, lipids need lipases, and proteins need proteases. These and other enzymes are present in milk as it comes from the animal. Lactose needs lactase to make it available. Lactase is not in the milk. It is produced and utilized in the intestines by the action of bacteria, e.g., lactobacilli, lactococci, and lactobifids. These beneficial bacteria are present in abundance in fresh unprocessed milk. Enzyme activity is generally maximized at body temperature.

Vitamins help control the metabolic processes. Milk provides many vitamins. Vitamins A and D are fat-soluble vitamins that work synergistically. Both are necessary to fulfill their individual nutritional tasks. They occur naturally together in milk. Vitamin D, essential for bone health, is associated with suppression of osteoporosis. Vitamin A is critical for immune function and the health of the eyes. Vitamin B-12 is found in animal foods. There is a significant amount of vitamin B-12 in milk. It plays a key role in folate metabolism, which prevents spina bifida in the developing fetus. B vitamins, especially niacin, are important for the normal functioning of many enzymes in the body and are involved in the metabolism of sugars and fatty acids.

Antioxidants can slow or even prevent cellular damage. Vitamins A and E and the mineral, selenium, are antioxidants that are present in milk in sufficient amounts to function appropriately. Selenium aids the body in manufacturing CoQ-10, (coenzyme) an enzyme that is specific for heart muscle health. Vitamin K-2 (menaquinone) is the form of the K vitamin found in milk. Mammals make K-2 from K-1 which is found in plants (phylloquinone), and is also made by the bacteria that line the human gastrointestinal tract. Some studies indicate that Vitamin K helps in maintaining strong bones in the elderly. Calcium cannot be assimilated without vitamin K. Vitamin K also plays an important role in blood clotting.

Whole milk has a balance of nutrients that are provided in a convenient form that is adaptable to many uses and, for most people, pleasant in taste. The nutritional value of milk is optimized by using whole, full-fat milk.

3. What are the additional benefits of milk fresh from the cow?

Milk fresh from the cow is a complete, living, functional food. Although we have looked at the numerous nutritional components of milk in the previous two questions, the full benefits of milk are only realized when all of these components function as a complex, interdependent, and balanced process. Included here are components that are not nutrients, although some do contribute indirectly to nutritional processes.

These components include:

Enzymes
Enzymes are specialized proteins produced in cells that link, break-up, or accelerate chemical reactions. They are considered catalysts because they are not consumed during the processes they control.

Intrinsic (Indigenous) Enzymes in Milk
There are many enzymes that exist naturally in fresh milk, known as intrinsic enzymes. Some intrinsic enzymes actively participate in the breakdown of components of milk, others break down the products of other enzymatic activity, still others have antimicrobial, and/or antiviral activity. As an example, milk, as a complete and adequate food for the newborn calf, contains nearly all of the necessary enzymes to make milk bioavailable. Some enzymes in the newborn calf's digestive tract are also active in making the components of milk bioavailable.

The entire process is complex and designed to function as an integrated system. It is this integrated system that is so important to the newborn calf during the rapid, crucial, and elaborate development that occurs in the weeks after birth. During this time the newborn's only intake is milk, providing the adequate amount of water and supplemented with air.

A partial list of well characterized intrinsic enzymes contained naturally in fresh milk includes:

• Acid Phosphate	• Aldolase	• Alkaline Phosphatases
• Amylase	• β-N-acetylglucosaminidase	• Catalase
• Esterases	• Glucose oxidase	• Glutathione peroxidase
• γ-Glutamyl transferase	• Lactoperoxidase	• Lipoprotein Lipase
• Lysozymes	• Phospholipase	• Proteinases, including
• Ribonuclease	• Sulphydry oxidase	plasmin and cathepsin
• Superoxide dismutase	• Xanthine oxidase	• Xanthine oxidoreductus

The enzymes found in milk can be large and complex, such as catalase, below:

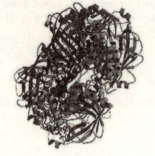

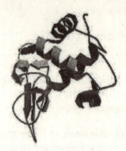

Others like the lysozymes are small and simple

*3D images are from the International Protein Database

Extrinsic Enzymes
Extrinsic Enzymes are enzymes that are made by microorganisms in milk, not produced by the mammary glands. These enzymes may be active in the milk or within the microorganisms themselves.

There are many such enzymes and they are very complex. Some of the specific enzymes are similar to those in the list of intrinsic enzymes. These enzymes are variable, depending on which specific bacteria are present in the milk. For the most part these enzymes participate in the breakdown of milk components to enable utilization by the microorganisms, but they also participate in the processes of bioavailability in the intestinal tract.

Because this list of enzymes is so variable and extensive, it is not practical to list them all here.

Immune System Enhancers
- Activation and enhancement of the innate immune system in newborns; these are nonspecific mechanisms that resist pathogens and toxins by interfering with their ability to cause infection.

- Triggering cell-mediated immune mechanisms; this system works by activating specific-response white blood cells to attack new and recurrent exposure to pathogens.

- Stimulation of specific immune reactions; this mechanism reacts in response to antigens by producing antibodies.

- Other specific immune active components: Compliment, Immunoglobulins (IgM, IgA, IgG), and Gamma Interferon

Cellular Elements
Bovine phagocytes and white blood cells in milk continue to be active within the digestive tract until they die, within days or weeks.

Many of the cellular elements measured in the Somatic Cell Count test of healthy cows, are exfoliated lining cells that release lysozymes when they are killed in the gastrointestinal tract as part of the normal digestive process. These lysozymes non-specifically attack microorganisms.

Additional Antibacterial Components
Digestion produces free fatty acids with bactericidal (kill bacteria) effects (medium-chain and short-chain fatty acids).

- Bacteriocins – Nisin, colicins, etc., are produced by beneficial microorganisms. There is a growing list of bacteriocins, compounds with bactericidal or bacteriostatic (inhibits bacteria) activity, produced by bacteria commonly found in fresh milk. Bacteriocins can be extremely specific or more general in their attack on other microorganisms.

- Mucins – Some pathogens rely on their ability to adhere to the intestinal cells in order to cause illness. Mucins are glycoproteins normally present on mucosal surfaces, including the intestines. The most studied mucin in milk is MUCI, which has been shown to adhere to bacteria and interfere with their ability to adhere to intestinal cells.

- Microorganisms that suppress pathogens by competitive mechanisms:
  o Compete for nutrients
  o Compete for intestinal attachment sites necessary for some pathogens to produce illness
  o Compete by limiting colonization of less robust microorganisms (this is also called competitive inhibition), such as pathogens

- Lactoferrin (iron binding glycoprotein that scavenges iron from the environment) – It has well documented bacteriostatic and bactericidal activity.

- Lactoperoxidase system – The system consists of the enzyme lactoperoxidase, with cofactors, thiocyanate and hydrogen peroxide. The complete functional system is naturally present in fresh milk. This is a potent antimicrobial system approved internationally to preserve milk, by adding more of the two cofactors, in locations where refrigeration is not practical.

- Lysozymes – Different forms of this enzyme are present in all cells, in a sequestered location. When cells are damaged, their store of lysozymes is released. Lysozymes have broad and effective antibacterial activity. Lysozymes are present in free form in fresh milk and are also released from the breakdown of bovine cells present in the milk.

- Xanthine oxidoreductase – Besides its role in nutrition, this enzyme augments intestinal defenses against pathogens by producing several reactive by-products.

Beneficial Microorganisms

There are large numbers of different bacteria present in fresh milk. Some of these are included in the Standard Plate Count test, while others do not grow under those culture conditions and so are not counted as a part of the test. Both the total numbers and the diversity of bacterial types (genus and species) are variable. Most of these bacteria are beneficial. (Some people would characterize these as probiotics; however, in the ever-evolving definition of probiotics, this term is currently confined to products in which beneficial microorganisms are added. Therefore, we will describe them as beneficial bacteria.)

As mentioned above, some of these beneficial bacteria have mechanisms for suppressing pathogens. A few of the best-known beneficial bacteria in fresh milk include:

- E. coli
  (the vast majority of E. coli is beneficial and naturally formed in our large intestines – the O157:H7 sub-type is one of the rare exceptions)

- Lactococci

- Lactobacilli

- Bifidobacteria

There are numerous other, mostly anaerobic, microorganisms, i.e., microorganisms that live without oxygen, that participate in the digestion of food and the assimilation of nutrients. Nearly all of these organisms enter milk from colonies that become established in the distal portions of the mammary gland passageways. It is probable that the specific genus and species vary between different cows over time, and depending on the environment.

Folate Binding Protein

Protein that assists in the uptake of folate in the intestine.

Vitamin-Cofactors, Promoters or Enablers
Some of the trace elements present in milk are essential to vitamin activity, such as carotenes.

Prebiotics
Unlike probiotics, prebiotics are recognized as anything that promotes the growth and activity of beneficial microorganisms. Therefore, milk is inherently a prebiotic since it contains lactose and numerous other components that can be utilized by beneficial bacteria. One specific prebiotic factor present in fresh milk is lactoferrin which, interestingly, is well known as an antibacterial agent but also promotes the growth of bifidobacteria.

Hormones
These are nearly all specifically bovine hormones, but there is evidence that they exert some influence prior to their inactivation. The amount of each of these hormones tends to vary during the normal reproductive cycle of the cow, as well as during the seasons of the year. The more common hormones include:

- Bovine growth hormone

- Bovine estrogens

- Bovine calcitonin

- Insulin-like growth factor-I (IGF-1)

- Bovine prolactin

- Bovine thyroid stimulating hormone

Vitamin B-12
There is a significant amount of vitamin B-12 in fresh milk. This vitamin is not present in plant foods and is a key to folate metabolism.

Trace Minerals
Specific trace elements are necessary as cofactors for many critical enzymes. The presence and amount of trace minerals is a function of dietary intake of the milk-producing animal. Essential trace minerals in milk include:
Iron, copper, zinc, manganese, cobalt, iodine, chromium, selenium, and molybdenum.

Others
- Freshness – Freshness provides enhanced ability to produce products from milk, such as:
  - Cream, Butter, Ghee (Indian clarified butter)

  - Curds & Whey products, e.g., soft cheeses

Report of Michigan Fresh Unprocessed Whole Milk Workgroup

- Cultured products such as cheeses, kefir, yogurt, cultured butter, and crème fraîche, etc.

  o Some of these rely on microorganisms and communities of microorganisms present in fresh milk that participate in the natural culturing of milk under controlled conditions.

  o Others are produced by using starters, such as for specific cheeses. These starters work best in milk that is less than two days old.

- Taste – Taste is rated high on beneficial values of fresh milk. It is naturally variable, mostly a function of feed, including types of forage, other added foods, and the animal breed. Seasonal variation is particularly noticeable. Geographic location is often responsible for specific, much sought-after tastes.

- Viscosity/Body – Viscosity is an important beneficial value, influenced by the fat content, aggregation of fats, and the interactions of proteins.

- Color – Color is variable depending on the fat content and the nature of forage, particularly on the amount of fresh, rapidly-growing grasses.

- Lactoferrin - Included above as an antibacterial property. Its ability to accumulate bioavailable iron is also a benefit.

- Overcoming the symptoms of lactose intolerance – Many people with professionally diagnosed lactose intolerance do not have the symptoms of this condition, even when consuming large amounts of fresh milk.

- Enhancement of mother's breast milk quality by including fresh milk in her diet.

- Fibrinolysis system components – Particularly important in the newborn, whose systems for combating inappropriate clotting have not developed fully.

- Reduction in asthma and allergic rhinitis – Numerous well controlled studies have shown the independent effect of drinking fresh milk to reduce asthma and childhood rhinitis in general, and specifically in childhood allergic rhinitis.

- Beneficial in some autistic children.

- Anti-stiffness/Anti-arthritis factor – Wurzen factor found in butterfat.

- Risk Reduction of Metabolic Syndrome – Increasing the consumption of milk and other dairy products may reduce metabolic syndrome (MetS); a

Report of Michigan Fresh Unprocessed Whole Milk Workgroup

report states that drinking a pint of milk daily is associated with a 62% risk reduction for MetS.

- Medical treatments using fresh milk – The "Raw Milk Diet" has a 150-year-old history. It was used in the Mayo Clinic and by others, and is currently practiced in Europe.

- Functional Medicine – The increased use of prebiotics, probiotics, and fresh milk to treat a variety of intestinal disorders.

- Intact milk fat globules are surrounded by a lipoprotein membrane. This membrane maintains the globule, resists metabolism and contains some of the enzymes and beneficial factors listed above.

4. What is the impact of pasteurization on the value of fresh unprocessed whole milk?

(Refer to Question 1. **What is the nutritional value of milk?** Question 2. **Going beyond the Nutrition Fact Label**, and Question 3. **What are the additional benefits of milk fresh from the cow?**)

Pasteurization is defined in the 2007 Grade "A" Pasteurized Milk Ordinance (PMO) as follows:
The terms "pasteurization", "pasteurized" and similar terms shall mean the process of heating every particle of milk, or milk product, in properly designed and operated equipment to one (1) of the temperatures given in the following chart and held continuously at, or above, that temperature for at least the corresponding specified time:

Temperature	Time
63°C (145°F)	30 minutes
72°C (161°F)	15 seconds
89°C (191°F)	1.0 seconds
90°C (194°F)	0.5 seconds
94°C (201°F)	0.1 seconds
96°C (204°F)	0.05 seconds
100°C (212°F)	0.01 seconds

Report of Michigan Fresh Unprocessed Whole Milk Workgroup

The term "Ultra-Pasteurization" when used to describe a dairy product means that the product has been thermally processed at, or above, 138°C (280°F) for at least two (2) seconds, either before or after packaging, so as to produce a product which has an extended shelf life under refrigerated conditions. (Refer to Code of Federal Regulations – 21CFR 131.3)

In addition to these time and temperature requirements for heating milk and milk products, the PMO requires that the equipment used to pasteurize and ultrapasteurize milk be properly designed, operated, and tested. These requirements are specified in PMO Item 16p, Appendix H and Appendix I.

All effects of pasteurization are variable, depending on temperature and time. There are many standards for pasteurization depending on the product being produced and the intended qualities of the end product. In addition, the components of milk differ greatly, and making different dairy products requires different levels of heat treatment and protein denaturation.

Impact on Proteins
Proteins are incrementally denatured by heat. With lower heat treatment levels, complex proteins with three-dimensional configuration are altered. With higher heat treatment levels, the primary shape and bonds are altered. At very high heat levels, there are destructive chemical changes.

The casein proteins themselves have been shown to be relatively heat stable. However, the actual bioavailability of the casein proteins is far more complicated. There are a large number of different casein proteins (as many as 1,000). These are "packaged" in the large and complex physical structure, the micelle. Individual micelles contain a variable mixture of these different caseins. The micelle functions as a reservoir of nutritionally important proteins; all of the essential amino acids combine to make up the different caseins, in a structure that is critical in the physical properties of milk, altering the enzymatic digestion of the proteins and affecting the movement through the intestine. The food industry is well aware that casein micelles are altered within the range of pasteurization time and temperatures, changing the way milk behaves when used to produce a variety of dairy products. Furthermore, the micelles contain both calcium and phosphorus, internalized in association with the proteins in specific concentrations and in physical forms, facilitating availability during digestion. It is well recognized that heating milk in the range of pasteurization alters the physical properties of the micelles. With heating, the whey proteins become bound to the micelles.

Whey proteins denature more readily, particularly the immunoglobulins.

Impact on Carbohydrates
Lactose undergoes the Maillard reaction, the chemical binding of sugar to protein also commonly known as the browning effect, which progresses as temperature is increased. This affects color and taste.

Impact on Fats
This is complex as changes to the fat globules, specifically the membranes, are caused by both heat and homogenization. Of all the milk constituents, the milk fat globule is the most drastically altered by the combination of pasteurization and homogenization.

Impact on Minerals
The minerals themselves are not affected by heat. However, what they are bound to is. For example, calcium and phosphorus are contained within the structure of the micelles and, thus, their intestinal absorption is affected by the heat treatment level.

Table – Impact of Heat, Temperature and Time

The table below summarizes broadly and in a qualitative manner the impact of heat, temperature, and time on the various nutritional components of fresh unprocessed whole milk. (Refer to Topic 2, Question 3. **What are the additional benefits of milk fresh from the cow?**)

NAME	EFFECTS OF HEAT, TEMPERATURE AND TIME
Intrinsic Enzymes	Some inactivation: Inactivation levels are extremely variable, from total inactivation (alkaline phosphate) to almost no effect (lysozymes)
Extrinsic Enzymes	Most bacteria are killed, so are not available as sources of extrinsic enzymes. More complex, as killing bacteria through heat doesn't necessarily eliminate all enzymes.
Immune System Enhancers Activation and enhancement of newborn innate immune system	To the extent that pasteurization kills most bacteria, they would not be present to trigger a newborn infant's innate immunity system.
Triggering cell-mediated immune mechanisms	Killed Cell-mediated immune mechanisms rely on living somatic cells, but pasteurization kills those cells, cancelling out that effect
Stimulation of immune reactions	Some denaturization Heat denatures protein in immunoglobulins, causing them to lose their ability to stimulate immune reactions
Other specific immune components	Variable All components are affected differently because they are chemically very different
Cellular Elements	Killed All living somatic cells, including bovine phagocytes and white blood cells, are killed by pasteurization

NAME	EFFECTS OF HEAT, TEMPERATURE AND TIME
Additional Antibacterial Components, Bacteriocins, Mucins	Variable effects Class of bacteriocins are removed, since the bacteria that produce them are killed. Mucins may be affected.
Microorganisms	Mostly killed
Lactoferrin	Some denaturization
Lactoperoxidase System	System rendered ineffective The enzyme itself isn't particularly affected, but it doesn't work without its cofactors, thiocyanate and hydrogen peroxide, making the system ineffective
Lysozymes	Little to no effect. Lysozymes are heat resistant, but killing bacteria and cells releases lysozymes, increasing the amounts overall.
Xanthine oxidoreductase	Activity is reduced Due to damage of the cellular membrane
Beneficial Organisms	Mostly killed
Pathogenic Organisms	Mostly Killed
Folate Binding Protein	Folate utilization reduced Folate itself is not particularly affected, but the protein that assists in uptake is denatured by heat

NAME	EFFECTS OF HEAT, TEMPERATURE AND TIME
Vitamin-Cofactors, Promoters or Enablers	Variable Amount of trace elements are not particularly affected by heat, but other cofactors may be.
Prebiotics	Value diminished
Hormones	The Workgroup has not found any available data on effect of heat and time on hormones in milk.
Vitamin B-12	The Workgroup is not aware of any effects
Trace Minerals	The Workgroup is not aware of any effects

OTHER ATTRIBUTES	EFFECTS OF HEAT, TEMPERATURE AND TIME
Taste, Viscosity/Body and Colour	Affected
Lactose Intolerance	Heating does not affect the level of lactose in milk. Although there are reports that many people with lactose intolerance do not experience symptoms when drinking fresh unprocessed whole milk, the Workgroup does not know if this affect is the result of pasteurization
Fibrinolysis	The Workgroup is unaware of any effects
Enhancement of Mother's Breast Milk from drinking Milk	The Workgroup does not have available information or studies on the effect of the nutritional value of breast milk to a mother who is consuming pasteurized milk

OTHER ATTRIBUTES	EFFECTS OF HEAT, TEMPERATURE AND TIME
Asthma and Allergic Rhinitis	The reduction of asthma and allergic rhinitis in children when raw milk is consumed is well documented. However, studies have not specifically determined if this is the effect of heating or of some other difference between FUW milk and commercial pasteurized milk.
Autism	The Workgroup does not know what the cause is, or if applying heat and time to milk affects autism
Arthritis	The Workgroup does not know what the cause is, or if applying heat and time to milk affects arthritis
Risk Reduction of Metabolic Syndrome	The Workgroup does not know what the cause is, or if applying heat and time to milk affects these.
Medical Treatments	The Workgroup does not know what the cause is, or if applying heat and time to milk affects these.
Functional Medicine	Beneficial bacteria are reduced by heat, so prebiotics and probiotics are affected
Intact Milk Fat Globules	Some denaturization of the milk fat globule membranes

Report of Michigan Fresh Unprocessed Whole Milk Workgroup

5.   What is the impact of homogenization on the value of fresh unprocessed whole milk?

The purpose of homogenization is to decrease the size of the fat globules to prevent a cream line and create a more uniform product. Fat globules are decreased by mechanical disruption.

Homogenization became standard practice because it made fluid milk easier to standardize and removed the cream line as a marketing property. In practice, homogenization is not performed without pasteurization because homogenized milk rapidly becomes rancid.

Homogenization is a physical action that substantially reduces the size of the milk fat globules. In the process, the complex lipoprotein membrane that surrounds the native fat globules is disrupted. This membrane is biologically active, containing many enzymes and a variety of active protein and mucin molecules. One of the critical functions of the membrane is to protect the internal fats from premature digestion. The smaller globules become enveloped by other proteins, the surface area becoming considerably increased as the globules are reduced in size, and there is not enough of the fragmented native membrane to complete the coating. The substituted proteins (mostly caseins) are not as effective in protecting the contained fats.

6.   Assuming that all milk is not the same, what do production and management practice have to do with fresh unprocessed whole milk's nutritional value, pathogens, color, taste, etc.?

Healthy Cows Provide Quality Milk

Pasture-Based Production Practices
There is evidence that properly managed pasture-based production practices improve the quality of milk. For example, cows that are pasture-based on primarily mixed grasses produce milk that is higher in CLA, beta-carotene, and fatty acids. A diverse grass/clover mix is best, and it does make a difference what types of grass mixes are used and how the pasture is managed. When cows are not on pasture, the fatty acids and vitamins in the milk decrease. A mixture of hay and fibrous grains are good winter feed for animals that are otherwise pastured. Whereas younger grasses have a higher protein content and produce more CLAs, mature grasses provide more minerals which are important to reproductive health.

A rule of thumb for animals in Michigan is one cow per acre of pasture. Thus, pastures must be managed carefully and actively, and with an eye on long term sustainability to produce high quality milk.

Report of Michigan Fresh Unprocessed Whole Milk Workgroup

Feeds and Grains
The content of feed, and changes in feeding, affect taste and color of milk. Proper management of fermented feeds reduces animal health risks.

Soil Quality
Soil and manure management practices have an effect on nutrient availability in soils which, in turn, has an effect on the nutrient composition of grasses and other feeds. This affects the nutritional quality of milk such as CLA, beta-carotene, and fatty acids. Additionally, the way soil and manure are managed has an effect on plant composition, soil microflora, and the presence of plant disease – causing organisms in the soil. All of these factors affect the nutrient value of the feed that the cows consume and, hence, the health of the cows.

Organic matter with appropriate humus content is an essential component of a healthy soil system. Building the system depends on the quality of the humus in the soil and the application of manure or other organic matter sources over time. Decomposition in these systems relies on aerobic activity, which converts organic matter into humus. Soils that are building organic matter tend to have more beneficial organisms, which help build beneficial soil microflora.

While anaerobic liquid manure systems are prevalent on dairy farms in Michigan, aerobic systems appear to produce manure that is more complimentary to soil quality. Key nutrients such as nitrogen (N) and potassium (K), are more easily managed in aerobic and grazing systems. These nutrients must be managed via application rates; too much of these two nutrients will cause an overfeeding of the plants, disrupting plant metabolism and, as a result, the nutritional value to the cows.

Variation is part of the value of fresh unprocessed whole milk
The taste/flavor and color of milk naturally varies according to breed of animal and what they are fed. These variations can be affected by farm management practices, which consumers of FUW milk accept and appreciate.

- Whole milk has a higher butterfat content. Fat plays the primary role in carrying the flavor of milk.

  A satisfying and pleasant richness is a characteristic of FUW milk. The more frequently a cow is milked, the lower the fat content per milking.

- Temporary variations in the taste of milk can also occur with a change of seasons and feeding patterns. There can be incidental unpleasant tastes resulting when a cow eats certain weeds (e.g. wild mustard, garlic, and wild onions) just before milking or when she is sick or in the very late part of her lactation cycle. Odors in cow housing and milking environments can cause off-flavors in the milk.

Report of Michigan Fresh Unprocessed Whole Milk Workgroup

- The color of the milk changes noticeably in the spring when cows are primarily eating green growing grass; it becomes cream-colored because of the increased levels of beta carotene in the butterfat.

7. What is the impact of consumer preferences on production and management practices of fresh unprocessed whole milk?

In a system in which consumers interact directly with the dairy farmer, some farm management choices are influenced by special consumer demands. There is no defined set of standards; however, based on discussions with the MI Fresh Milk Council, Michigan consumers, and farmers providing FUW milk, there are some common preferences:

- They want the way the farm is managed to be dedicated to the production of milk intended to be consumed without processing, and farmers that welcome inspection of their operations.

- They want the cows to have free access to pasture, not raised and maintained in confinement.

- They want the cows fed forage, preferably pastured on grasses.

- They want the milk to be in a fresh natural state without processing, e.g. unpasteurized, not homogenized, and with nothing removed and nothing added.

- They expect high butterfat content.

- They want the animals to be well cared for.

- They specifically do not want feed that includes genetically engineered crop products, any soy, or by-products like brewer grain, beet pulp, or cotton seed.

- They do not want any pharmaceuticals used to enhance milk production.

- They prefer no use of chemical fertilizers, herbicides, or pesticides on the farm.

- They are willing to pay for quality.

- They are willing to go out of their way to get the milk.

Report of Michigan Fresh Unprocessed Whole Milk Workgroup

References

This is the full link to the Haug article used in all of Topic 2 Values and Benefits. [Cited url: http://www.pubmedcentral.nih.gov/articlerender.fcgi?artid=2039733 Revised url: https://lipidworld.biomedcentral.com/articles/ 10.1186/1476-511X-6-25]

Question 1: What is the nutritional value of milk?

- "Comparison of Nutritional Content of Various Milks", David B. Fankhauser, PhD, Professor University of Cincinnati, Cincinnati, Ohio. Cited url: http://biology.clc.uc.edu/fankhauser/Cheese/milk_content.htm [Revised url: https://fankhauserblog.wordpress.com/tag/microbiology/page/3/]

- "Daily Values - A guide for Nutrient Labeling", University of Texas. Cited url: http://www.utexas.edu/courses/ntr3ll/nutinfo.dvalues.html [no longer available, redirected to: https://www.utexas.edu/]

- Dietary Supplement Fact Sheet: Calcium" (Chart) 2005. The National Institutes of Health Office of Dietary Supplements

- "Calcium and Milk" 2004. Harvard University School of Public Health

- "Nutrition Information - Whole Milk" Chart. Cited url: http://www.nutritiondata.com/facts [no longer available, redirected to: https://www.self.com/]

- *Dairy Chemistry and Physics*. Douglas Goff, PhD, Professor of Food Science, University of Guelph, Toronto, Canada. Cited url: http://www.foodsci.uoguelph.ca/dairyedu/chem.html [Revised url, ebook: https://books.lib.uoguelph.ca/dairyscienceandtechnologyebook/]

- "Building Strong Bones: Calcium Information for Health Care Providers". The National Institute of Child Health and Human Development (NICHD).

- "Milk's Unique Nutrient Package", The National Dairy Council.

Books

- *MILK: Its Remarkable Contribution to Human Health and Well-Being* by Stuart Patton, PhD, Professor Emeritus, Food Science, Pennsylvania State University, Transaction Publisher, NJ 2004

- *On Food and Cooking, the Science and Lore of the Kitchen* by Harold McGee, Chapter 1. Milk and Dairy Products. Scribner, NY, 2004 http://www.curiouscook.com

---

Report of Michigan Fresh Unprocessed Whole Milk Workgroup

Question 2: Going beyond the Nutrition Facts Label – What other nutritional values should we be considering?

- "Bovine milk in human nutrition – a review". Table 1: Additional nutrients in milk and their main health effects, Anna Haug. et al. Lipids Health Dis. 2007: 6:25 Published online 2007 September 25. doi: 10.1186/1476-5llx-6-25. [Cited url: http://www.pubmedcentral.nih.gov/articlerender.fcgi?artid=2039733 Revised url, for Table 1: https://lipidworld.biomedcentral.com/articles/10.1186/1476-511X-6-25/tables/1]

- Nutrient Values and Weight – Milk, whole 3.5% milk fat (chart), USDA. [Cited url, no longer accessible: www.nal.usda.gov/fnic/foodcomp/cgi-bin/list_nut_edit.pl]

- "Understanding Milk's Bioactive Components: A Goal for the Genomics Toolbox" by Robert E. Ward and J. Bruce German, Journal of Nutrition, Vol. 134: 962S-967S; 2004

- "Milk and dairy consumption, diabetes and the metabolic syndrome: the Caerphilly prospective study" by P.C. Elwood, J.E. Pickering, A.M. Fehily, Journal of Epidemiology and Community Health Vol. 61, pages 695-698

Books

- *The Family Cow* by Dirk van Loon, Storey Books

- *Keeping a Family Cow* by Joann S. Grohman, Coburn Press

Question 3: What are the additional benefits of milk fresh from the cow?

<u>Enzymes –</u>
- "Indigenous enzymes in milk: Overview and historical aspects - Part 1 and 2" by P.F. Fox, A.L. Kelly; a thorough review with extensive references presented in the first Symposium on Indigenous Enzymes in Milk and later published in the International Dairy Journal, 2006

<u>Mucin –</u>
- "Some Practical Implications of the Milk Mucins", Stuart Patton, PhD, Professor Emeritus of food science at Pennsylvania State University; Review paper given at a symposium at Michigan State Univ. in 1998 and published in the Journal of Dairy Science. 1999.

Trace Minerals –
- "Adequacy of Trace Minerals in Bovine Milk for Human Consumption", by Donald Oberleas, PhD and Ananda S. Prasad, MD, PhD, The American Journal of Clinical Nutrition. Vol. 22, No.2, Feb. 1969, p 196-199

Allergies & Asthma –
- "Which aspects of the farming lifestyle explain the inverse association with childhood allergy?" by Michael R. Perkin, MSc and David P. Strachan, MD, Division of Community Health Sciences of St George's University of London, London, UK Journal Allergy Clinical Immunology 2006; 117:1374-81

- "Unpasteurized milk: health or hazard?" by M. R. Perkin, Division of Community Health Sciences of St George's University of London, London, UK Clinical and Experimental Allergy, 2007; 37, 6227-630

- "Inverse association of farm milk consumption with asthma and allergy in rural and suburban populations across Europe", The PARSIFAL study group (European Union grant). Journal compilation © 2006 Blackwell Publishing Ltd, Clinical and Experimental Allergy, 37:661 670

Metabolic Syndrome –

- Dairy May Protect Against Metabolic Syndrome" from: "Milk and Dairy Consumption, Diabetes and the Metabolic Syndrome: the Caerphilly Prospective Study" Wales study in 2007 of 20-year follow-up by P. C. Elwood, J. E. Pickering, M. Fehily. Journal of Epidemiology and Community Health, Vol. 61, pages 695-698

Questions 4, 5: What is the impact of pasteurization on the value of fresh unprocessed whole milk? What is the impact of homogenization on the value of fresh unprocessed whole milk?
- Dairy Science and Technology, Second edition CRC Taylor and Francis 2006, P. Walstra, T.M. Jan, T.M. Wouters, and Geurts. Chapter 7. Heat Treatment and Chapter 9. Homogenization.

- Interview with Dr. John Partridge, Professor at Michigan State University (MSU) Food Science & Human Nutrition

- Grade A Pasteurized Milk Ordinance (PMO) of 2007 [Cited url: http://www.michigan.gov/documents/mda/MDA_DP_07PMOFinal_251324_7.pdf Revised url, 2017 ed.: https://www.michigan.gov/mdard/-/media/Project/Websites/mdard/documents/food-dairy/dairy/grade_a_pasteurized_milk_ordinance.pdf]

Question 6: Assuming that all milk is not the same, what do production and management practice have to do with fresh unprocessed whole milk's nutritional value, pathogens, color, taste, etc.?

- Interview with Edwin Blosser, Midwest Bio-Systems

- Interview with Dr. George Bird, Professor of Entomology at MSU Interview with Joe Scrimger, Bio-Systems

- Interview with Warnke Family, Warnke's Emerald Acres Farm

- "Outbreaks associated with unpasteurized milk and soft cheese: an overview of consumer safety". Food Protection Trends, April 2009

Question 7: What is the impact of consumer preferences on production and management practices of fresh unprocessed whole milk?

- *Safe Handling* – Consumers' Guide – Preserving the Quality of Fresh Unprocessed Whole Milk by Peggy Beals, RN

Topic 3

Risks

1. What are the risks for fresh unprocessed whole milk, including all types of risks, such as adverse consequences, intolerance, and allergens?

2. Where do these risks originate?

Summary

Approved August 23, 2011

Topic 3 – Risks

Introduction

The Workgroup follows a set of topics and within each topic a set of questions. For Topic 3 – Risk, the Workgroup combined: Question 1. **What are the risks for fresh, unprocessed, whole milk, including all types of risks, such as pathogens, adverse consequences, intolerance, and allergens with** Question 2. **Where do these risks originate?**

They reviewed each of the four (4) groups of bacteria that are considered important causes of current foodborne illnesses in this country: *Campylobacter jejuni, Listeria monocytogenes,* Salmonella, and the O157:H7 subtype of *Escherichia. coli.* They also reviewed the bacteria that cause human illnesses and have historically dominated public health concerns. They also reviewed information on non-infectious adverse reactions to milk.

The summary includes the following sections:

- for each of the four pathogens a **Milkborne Bacterial Human Pathogen Summary** (outlining a description, types of diseases in animals and humans, and information on outbreaks)

- for each of the four pathogens a **Scenario for transmission to people** (which systematically outline patterns of spread of illness with emphasis on routes of transmission that pertain to milk consumption)

- A discussion of **Infectious Dose**

- A narrative on the illnesses of **Historical Interest**

- A discussion of the **Categories of Risk Other Than Infectious Disease for People Consuming Fresh Unprocessed Whole Milk (FUW Milk)**

- A **Table of Terms** - Recognizing that some of the terms used in the documents in Topic 3 might need explanation, the Workgroup developed a Table of Terms with a description (not dictionary definitions) to help the reader understand the terms as they are used in the context of the Summary on Risk. For the reader's convenience, the terms in the Table of Terms are highlighted in gray at their first use in each section. The Table of Terms begins on page 67.

Report of Michigan Fresh Unprocessed Whole Milk Workgroup

> *The Michigan Fresh Unprocessed Whole (FUW) Milk Workgroup Topic 3 – Risk discussion participants included Ted and Peggy Beals, Susan Esser, Katherine Fedder, Frank Fear, Rosanne Ponkowski, Joe Scrimger, John and Patti Warnke, Howard Straub and Elaine Brown.*

Milkborne Bacterial Human Pathogen Summaries

Campylobacter jejuni

Scientific Name: genus: Campylobacter **species:** jejuni **abbreviated:** *C. jejuni*

Recognized Subtypes within the species:
There are several commonly used systems of subtyping, with between 60 to 100 recognized subtypes using these different techniques. [1] [2] [3]

General
- Gram negative, rod-shaped, motile bacterium. The only natural habitat is the intestinal tract of many warm-blooded animals, but it is widespread in the natural environment when persistent animal fecal contamination occurs. Also common as a transient contaminant in home kitchens, water, and food manufacturing facilities.

- Easily cultured and detected when present in large numbers (such as in human diarrhea specimens). However, it is specifically difficult to culture from unpasteurized milk because of the multiple conditions listed below.

- Conditions that promote growth/survival: Optimal growth is within living cells. Growth is optimal at 108°F. Survival is best in warm, wet conditions.

- Conditions that inhibit growth/survival: Generally described as "fragile", this bacteria is sensitive to air (oxygen), drying, and acidic environments and grows poorly, if at all, at room temperatures. It does not grow well outside of warm-blooded animal hosts. It does not compete well with other bacteria, and isolation techniques are usually required to inhibit those other bacteria. The numbers decline over time in unprocessed milk, particularly when refrigerated or exposed to air. Unprocessed milk with other bacteria tends to become acidic, due to the growth of the other bacteria. Specific research on the fate of *Campylobacter jejuni*, isolated from human cases and inoculated into unpasteurized milk under laboratory conditions, documented inactivation over several days. [4]

Report of Michigan Fresh Unprocessed Whole Milk Workgroup

Disease Description

Animals
Present in healthy birds and other animal intestines (carrier state) but rarely causes disease.

Humans

- Acute gastroenteritis with diarrhea categorized as campylobacteriosis. Nearly all human infections are from *C. jejuni*, but a few are from *C. coli*.

- The most common foodborne illness in the U.S. with 2 million cases per year (1 illness per 150 people each year).

- Interval from consumption to symptoms is 3-5 days. Illness is usually self-limiting (recovery without antibiotics) lasting for 3-12 days. However, in untreated cases, individuals may continue to shed infectious bacteria for 7 weeks. A true persistent carrier state (colonizing in intestine without illness) in humans is rare.

- Because of huge numbers of bacteria present in diarrhea, culturing in the medical laboratory is a practical means of making the diagnosis.

- There are at least four virulence steps necessary for human illness: (1) adheres to intestinal cells; (2) grows in the intestine; (3) enters the cell and proliferates; (4) produces toxin.

- During 2009 there were 911 reported cases of campylobacter gastroenteritis in Michigan. Frequency of illnesses in humans is seasonal, the highest being in June, July, and August.

Category of Human Disease

- Causes acute enteritis with nausea, abdominal cramps, severe diarrhea, which may be bloody, and mild fever

- Infectious dose: from 500 to 10,000 virulent bacteria depending on foods consumed and health of the person

- Immunity results from frequent direct contact with farm animals.

Complications of Human Infection

Rare. A form of Guillain-Barré Syndrome occurs in about 1 out of 1,000 human cases of campylobacteriosis. This inflammatory neurologic syndrome has been associated with a number of other viral and bacterial infections.

Reservoir (potential source)

- Humans with campylobacter enteritis shed 1,000,000 bacteria per gram of diarrhea.

- All warm-blooded animals, particularly birds, become exposed in infancy and persist as carriers of campylobacter in their intestines throughout their lives.

- Chickens shed 1,000,000 or more colony-forming-units per gram (cfu/gram). [5]

- Water, contaminated from animal manure

- Cows whose intestines are temporarily colonized with *C. jejuni* shed comparatively low numbers in their feces. [6]

- Shedding directly from an infection into the milk does not occur.

- A study in rural Michigan found that poultry husbandry carried the greatest risk of human campylobacter enteritis. [7]

Food Implicated in Outbreaks

Surveys show that 20%-100% of retail chicken packages are contaminated. It is estimated that one drop of fluid from fresh packaged chicken contains an infectious dose.

Outbreaks

Most campylobacter foodborne outbreaks are limited to a few cases of illness; however, some outbreaks from contaminated water supplies have caused illness in thousands of people.

- Fresh unprocessed whole milk in Michigan 1999-2011 [8] – 36 illnesses

- Fresh unprocessed whole milk U.S. 1999-2011 [8] – Total 383 illnesses (average 31.9 per year)

- For all foods, estimated annual illnesses from Campylobacter spp. in the U.S., based on data collected in 2006-2008 [9] – 845,024

Numbered Specific References

Unless referenced separately, most of the comments are from the FDA "Bad Bug Book" Foodborne Pathogenic Microorganisms and Natural Toxins Handbook.

Report of Michigan Fresh Unprocessed Whole Milk Workgroup

[Cited url: www.cfsan.fda.gov/-mow/chapl.html Revised url: https://www.fda.gov/food/foodborne-pathogens/bad-bug-book-second-edition]

[1] "Campylobacteriosis". Center for Infectious Disease Research and Policy. Academic Health Center University of Minnesota, 2008.

[2] "Assessing Health Benefits of Controlling Campylobacter in the Food Chain". European Food Safety Authority Scientific Colloquium Summary Report 12, 2008. Rome, Italy.

[3] Common Somatic O and Heat-Labile Serotypes among Campylobacter Strains from Sporadic Infections in the United States. Patton, et al, 1992. Journal of Clinical Microbiology; 31(6): 1525-1530. (CDC)

[4] Prevalence and Survival of Campylobacter jejuni in unpasteurized milk. Doyle and Roman. Applied and Environmental Microbiology 44 (5): 1154-1158, 1982.

[5] Campylobacter in primary animal production and control strategies to reduce the burden of human Campylobacteriosis. Wagenaar, et al. Rev. sci. tech. Off. int. Epiz. 2006, 25(2):581-594.

[6] Chronic shedding of Campylobacter species in beef cattle. Inglis, et al. 2004, Journal of Applied Microbiology 97:410-420.

[7] Risk Factors for Sporadic Campylobacter jejuni Infections in Rural Michigan: A Prospective Case - Control Study. Potter, Kaneene, Hall. American Journal of Public Health, 2003; 93 (12): 2118-2123.

[8] Illnesses enumerated for outbreaks were obtained from a comprehensive listing of incidents with official reports for the period, January 1, 1999 to March 30, 2011. All incidents were entered into the database from news releases and public reports from national and state agencies, media articles, published listings from public interest groups and litigation websites, scientific publications, as well as from personal information. Numbers displayed in the Pathogen Summary documents include both confirmed and presumed illnesses given in final reports without any evaluation of the way the officials made their determination. There is no judgment on the manner of the investigation nor on the strength of the conclusions. Only incidents within the U.S. were included, and only when the investigation specified consumption of fluid fresh unprocessed milk as the presumed source. Both cow and goat dairies that were specifically operated for the purpose of supplying fresh unprocessed milk to consumers were included.

[9] Foodborne Illness Acquired in the United States --- Major Pathogens, Elaine Scallan, R.M. Hoekstra, F.J. Angulo, R.V. Tauxe, M. Widdowson, S.L. Roy, J.J. Jones and P.M/ Griffin, Emerg. Infect. Dis. 2011. Table 2, pg. 16. Note that the numbers are specific for domestically acquired illnesses.

Listeria monocytogenes

Scientific Name: genus: listeria **species**: monocytogenes
abbreviated: *L. monocytogenes*

General

Gram positive, motile, small, rod-shaped bacterium. This organism is widely found in nature. In nature it multiplies under a broad range of conditions including -2 to 80°F, and in the presence or absence of oxygen. It is capable of survival over long intervals and under adverse conditions. Its ability to multiply and survive under adverse conditions (particularly refrigeration) gives it a competitive advantage.

However, growth is very slow with a doubling time of 1-2 days at 39°F. Some strains are able to form biofilms. Strains are remarkably stable, with one persisting in a processing plant for 12 years.

In addition to its presence in the environment, some subtypes are capable of entering living animal cells and altering their growth requirements, thus enabling them to rapidly multiply and spread between cells to cause illness.

Recognized Virulent Subtypes within the species

This is an extremely well-studied and complex organism. There are more than 13 documented serotypes using the H (flagellar) and O (somatic) characteristics. The commonly used serotyping (l/2a, l/2b, l/2c, 3a, etc.) are based on "O" antigens. Three lineages have been used to categorize this species, each with different patterns of serotypes and characteristic environmental niches.

Lineage	Isolates Primarily From:
I	Human Illness
II	Foods & Non-Human Illnesses
III	Animal & Some Human Illnesses

Most human illnesses are associated with the serotypes l/2a, l/2b and 4b. [1]

Disease Description

Perhaps best understood as an accidental pathogen in humans, but primarily a source of disease in a large number of non-human animals. [2]

Humans

There are several different disease patterns. Within individual outbreaks there is a dominant pattern.

Disease patterns:

1. Systemic: Spreads to organs in the body. In these cases, the virulent pathogen circulates in the blood (bacteremia). The most common locations for organ infections are: brain, liver, and the pregnant uterus. These illnesses tend to be severe, with hospitalization and mortality common.

2. Perinatal illnesses: The pregnant woman may have only a mild gastroenteritis or flu-like episode. However, if bacteria enter the blood stream, infection during pregnancy is most likely localized in the uterus, resulting in disease in the embryo, placenta, or newborn. The transmitted disease is often severe with high mortality.

3. Gastroenteritis: Mild, self-limiting illness.

- The infectious dose is extremely variable, ranging from 100 to 1,000,000, or higher, bacteria.[1]

- It is believed that many people (and animals) are occasionally exposed, some with very high doses, without evidence of illness. The incubation period in human illnesses varies from several days to many weeks.

- 98% of human illnesses are with serovars 1/2a, 1/2b and 4b

- The most common serotype virulent in humans with systemic listeriosis is 4b; the most associated with gastroenteritis is 1/2a.

- There are widely spaced outbreaks with many ill people, suggesting that there are epidemic clones.

- Most human cases, not related to pregnancy, are in adults and are caused by ingestion of contaminated food. Only 7% of cases occur in the healthy general public. The other cases have an underlying immunocompromizing condition (cancer, HIV/AIDS, immunosuppressant medications). Spread between humans is uncommon.

- Although of public health importance, "it appears that *L. monocytogenes* represents an opportunistic human pathogen and that human infections are likely to contribute little if anything to the ecological success or dispersal of *L. monocytogenes*". [2]

Classification of Illness Caused by *Listeria monocytogenes*

TYPE OF ILLNESS	MODE OF TRANS-MISSION	INFECTIOUS DOSE	SEVERITY	INCUBATION PERIOD
Skin Infection	Direct physical contact	Very High	Mild self-limiting	Several days
Neonatal Infection	Direct contact between mother and newborn, or other infected newborn	Unknown	Severe, usually central nervous system and, frequently, death	1-12 days
Pregnant Women	Foodborne	High	Mild flu-like symptoms or mild gastroenteritis; consequences to fetus or newborn is usually severe	Unknown
Non-Pregnant Adults	Foodborne	High	Mild, but in rare cases can be severe with hospitalization for systemic disease. May lead to death	1 day to months Mostly 3 to 4 weeks
Gastro-enteritis	Foodborne	Extremely High (10 000 000 organisms)	Vomiting, diarrhea, fever, often mild and self-limiting	1 or more days

Report of Michigan Fresh Unprocessed Whole Milk Workgroup

Animals

Predominately in <u>ruminant animals</u> (sheep, cattle, goats and, occasionally, pigs) but also in nonruminants, birds, fish, and reptiles. The pattern of disease is very similar to those described above for humans, except that in domestic ruminants, infection may spread through the herd and can be severe. Manure from cattle with listeriosis (circling disease) and from infected products-of-abortion contain very high concentrations of *L. monocytogenes*. And, as with humans, there is evidence that animals may be exposed without illness. Transient colonization is common. Incidence in cattle is reducing, generally attributed to awareness of risk from poorly managed silage (containing as many as 1,000,000 organisms per gram) as a major source of listeriosis.

Category of Pathogen - For all Animals

- Causing acute enteritis with nausea, abdominal cramps, and mild diarrhea.
- Causing systemic diseases localizing predominately in the liver, brain, and pregnant uterus.
- Uterine infections in pregnancy, resulting in infections of the embryo or newborn.

Complications of Human Infection

Hospitalization with the systemic disease is common. Death rate following systemic infections is high.

Reservoir

Widely found in the environment and animals. Has a competitive advantage in salty or cold environments. Although much is known about the growth and survival in various ecosystems, transmission and principal sources are poorly understood, perhaps because it has developed different mechanisms in different systems. It appears that *Listeria monocytogenes* represents an opportunistic human pathogen and that human infections are likely to contribute little, if anything, to the ecological success or dispersal of *Listeria monocytogenes*.

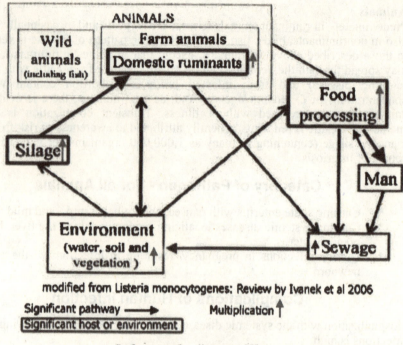

References for diagram. [3]

Foods Implicated in Human Outbreaks

Fresh, undamaged, or unprocessed foods do not support the growth of this organism.

By all measures, ready-to-eat meats (such as deli meats) are the most frequently associated with outbreaks. Contamination in these products occurs in the processing plant environment, including the processing equipment. Due to the association with processing environments, the list of implicated foods is very long, including processed meats such as pate, salami, hot dogs, processed fish, cheeses, processed vegetables, and salads. Specific foods associated with outbreaks are related to trends in food consumption and processing rather than to the individual foods themselves.

Foodborne human illness is mostly associated with those processed foods which ordinarily have a long shelf life at refrigerated temperatures.

Outbreaks for *Listeria monocytogenes:*

- Fresh unprocessed whole milk in Michigan 1999-2011 [4] - 0 illnesses

- Fresh unprocessed whole milk U.S. 1999-2011 [4] - 0 illnesses

- For all foods, estimated annual illnesses from Listeria monocytogenes in the U.S. based on data collected in 2006-2008 [5] – 1,591

General References

FDA "Bad Bug Book" Foodborne Pathogenic Microorganisms and Natural Toxins Handbook. [Cited url: https://www.fda.gov/food/foodsafety/foodborneillness/foodborneillnessfoodbornepathgensnaturaltoxins/badbugbook/ucm070064.htm Revised url: https://www.fda.gov/food/foodborne-pathogens/bad-bug-book-second-edition]

Advisory Committee on the Microbiological Safety of Food's Draft Report on Increased Incidence of Listeriosis in the UK. 2008

Epidemiological and Experimental Studies of Listeria Infection, with special reference to fecal excretion in ruminants, contamination of raw milk, presence in silage, and growth at low temperatures. Jaana Husu, [Definitive thesis and associated published articles; Helsinki, 1990]

Risk assessment of Listeria monocytogenes in ready-to-eat foods. Microbiological Risk Assessment Series 4. WHO/FAO, 2004

Numbered Specific References

[1] Wiedmann, M. Molecular Subtyping Methods for Listeria monocytogenes. J. of AOAC International 85(2):524-531. 2002

[2] Oliver, Wiedmann and Boor. Environmental Reservoir and Transmission into the Mammalian Host. Chapter 6 pp 122-148. In *Listeria monocytogenes: Pathogenesis and Host Response.* ed. Goldfine and Shen. Springer 2007

[3] Ivanek, R., et al. Listeria monocytogenes in Multiple Habitats and Host Populations: Review of Available Data for Mathematical Modeling. 2006. Foodborne Pathogens and Disease 3(4):319-336.

[4] Illnesses enumerated for outbreaks were obtained from a comprehensive listing of incidents with official reports for the period, January 1, 1999 to March 30, 2011. All incidents were entered into the database from news releases and public reports from national and state agencies, media articles, published listings from public interest groups and litigation websites, scientific publications, as well as from personal information. Numbers displayed in the Pathogen Summary documents

include both confirmed and presumed illnesses given in final reports without any evaluation of the way the officials made their determination. There is no judgment on the manner of the investigation nor on the strength of the conclusions. Only incidents within the U.S. were included, and only when the investigation specified consumption of fluid fresh unprocessed milk as the presumed source. Both cow and goat dairies that were specifically operated for the purpose of supplying fresh unprocessed milk to consumers were included.

[5] Foodborne Illness Acquired in the United States—Major Pathogens, Elaine Scallan, R.M. Hoekstra, F.J. Angulo, R.V. Tauxe, M.A. Widdowson, S.L. Roy, J.L. Jones and P.M. Griffin, Emerg. Infect. Dis. 2011. Table 2, pg. 16. Note that the numbers are specific for domestically acquired illnesses.

Salmonella

Scientific Name: genus: *Salmonella spp.*

General
Salmonella is a gram negative, rod-shaped, motile bacteria. Its normal habitat is the intestinal tract of many warm and cold-blooded animals. But with widespread fecal contamination, it can be found throughout the environment. It is also identified as a contaminant in water supplies, food manufacturing facilities, and domestic kitchens. It survives for long periods in the environment, but does not generally multiply in the environment. However, some animal feeds and processed foods that are high in protein can support their growth when not refrigerated. Salmonella does not compete well with other bacteria and is inhibited in acidic conditions. Studies indicate that the few serovars that cause disease in humans, and the equally small number that cause disease in cows, are distinctly different. Essentially, all of the subtypes of salmonella were initially discovered from illnesses in different animals. The general opinion is that this organism has, over time, "host adapted" to many animals.

Recognized Subtypes (Serovars)
Two species are generally listed: enterica and bongori. Enterica is divided into 6 subspecies: enterica, salamae, arizonae, diarizonae, indica, and houtenae. Most of the human public health interest is in the subtype, *Salmonella enterica* subtype enterica. [1]

Recognized Virulent Subtypes
Species have a confusing naming system, and many names have been derived from specific animals or disease outbreaks. Some species or named serovars contain human virulent strains. Although some serotype names imply specific animals, many are widely distributed in other animals, as well as the environment.

Salmonella enterica Typhi causes typhoid but, as the human disease has been controlled, this is not a significant pathogen in the U.S. today (See the History topic). There are more than 2,500 documented serotypes; of these only about 50 have been associated with human illness. Many different virulence factors have been identified. The virulence factors differ between subtypes, and sometimes even within specific serotypes. Even if a specifically named serotype has been associated with human illness, this does not mean that any strain of that particular named serotype, found in another animal or as a contaminant in food, is capable of causing illness in humans.

Disease Description

Animals
Most animals that are clinically ill with salmonella subtypes have gastroenteritis. Systemic infections and abortions are known to be associated with specific subtypes and animals. Like typhoid in humans, some of the named serotypes are a significant health threat in specific animals. There are "host-adapted" subtypes, most of which cause specific diseases in specific animal hosts. Such host-adapted subtypes commonly develop carrier states. The more generalized subtypes, isolated from many different animals, may cause severe illness in a specific animal host, but cause gastroenteritis in other animals. Most salmonella found in cows are long-term colonizers.

Humans
Salmonellosis is the most common bacterial foodborne illness in the U.S., occurring mostly as sporadic cases with acute gastroenteritis. The interval from consumption to symptoms is shorter than for other milkborne gastroenteritis (12 hours to several days). A human carrier state is recognized for typhoid which is host-adapted to humans. Some studies indicate a small number of people with non-typhoidal salmonella gastroenteritis become carriers. Among many of the named serovars isolated from humans somewhere in the world, only a few are seen with any frequency; most have not been isolated from humans for decades. Although the FDA gives an infectious dose of 15-20 cells for salmonella spp., a USDA review list of minimal infectious dose studies using human volunteers ranges from 100,000-1,000,000,000 for specific serovars. [2]

Category of Pathogen

Essentially all subtypes cause illness in some animals. Most cause a mild acute enteritis with nausea, abdominal cramps, and mild diarrhea that last for a short period and generally do not require treatment. However, specific subtypes cause severe systemic disease in specific animals.

Complications of Human Infection

Rare

Report of Michigan Fresh Unprocessed Whole Milk Workgroup

Reservoir

- All birds and many amphibians may shed large amounts of bacteria in feces
- Water, contaminated from animal sources
- Cattle and cows, temporarily colonized, shed low numbers in feces.
- Contaminated feed is a significant source of recolonization within herds.

Other Food Implicated in Outbreaks

Most human cases are from eggs, packaged fresh poultry, and meat and foods prepared from these items.

Outbreaks for Salmonella

- Fresh unprocessed whole milk in Michigan 1999- 2011 [3] – 0 illnesses
- Fresh unprocessed whole milk U.S. 1999-2011 [3] – Total 39 illnesses (average 3.3 per year)
- For all foods, estimated annual illnesses from Salmonella spp. in U.S based on data collected in 2006-2008 [4] –1,027,561

General References

FDA "Bad Bug Book" Foodborne Pathogenic Microorganisms and Natural Toxins Handbook. [Cited url: www.cfsan.fda.gov/-mow/chapI.html Revised url: https://www.fda.gov/food/foodborne-pathogens/bad-bug-book-second-edition]

Uzzau, et. al. 2000. Review: Host adapted serotypes of Salmonella enterica. Epidemiology and Infection 125:229-255

Numbered Specific References

[l] Semenov, 2008. Doctoral thesis: Ecology and modeling of Escherichia coli O157:H7 and Salmonella enterica serovars Typhimurium in cattle manure and soils.

[2] Kothary, M. and Babu, U. 2001. Infective Dose of Foodborne Pathogens in Volunteers: A Review. Journal of Food Safety 21: 49-73.

[3] Illnesses enumerated for outbreaks were obtained from a comprehensive listing of incidents with official reports for the period, January 1, 1999 to March 30, 2011. All incidents were entered into the database from news releases and public reports from national and state agencies, media articles, published listings from public interest groups and litigation websites, scientific publications, as well as from

personal information. Numbers displayed in the Pathogen Summary documents include both confirmed and presumed illnesses given in final reports without any evaluation of the way the officials made their determination. There is no judgment on the manner of the investigation nor on the strength of the conclusions. Only incidents within the U.S. were included, and only when the investigation specified consumption of fluid fresh unprocessed milk as the presumed source. Both cow and goat dairies that were specifically operated for the purpose of supplying fresh unprocessed milk to consumers were included.

[4] Foodborne Illness Acquired in the U.S. – Major Pathogens, Elaine Scallan, R.M. Hoekstra, F.J. Angulo, R.V. Tauxe, M. Widdowson, S.L. Roy, J.J. Jones and P.M. Griffin, Emerg. Infect. Dis. 201 l. Table 2, pg. 16. Note that the numbers are specific for domestically acquired illnesses.

Escherichia coli

Scientific Name: genus: Escherichia   **species:** coli   **abbreviated:** *E. coli*

General Description and Information
Gram negative, rod-shaped bacterium; many, but not all, are motile. It grows well in oxygen containing, or depleted, environments. Its natural habitat is the intestinal tract of most warm-blooded and some cold-blooded animals but, with fecal contamination, becomes widespread in the natural environment. *E. coli* can also be found as contaminants in domestic kitchens, water, and food manufacturing facilities. Optimal growth is at 99°F. Easily cultured and detected, however, due to the diversity of the bacteria, there is no universal growth media for laboratory isolation. It is widely publicized that *E. coli* grows extremely rapidly, doubling in less than half an hour. These growth rates are under laboratory conditions in optimal growth media and at 98.6°F.

Nearly all *E. coli* are benign and some are, in fact, extremely beneficial, participating in digestion and metabolism in the intestinal tract.

Recognized Subtypes Within the Species
There are a number of commonly used systems for distinguishing forms of *E. coli*, resulting in hundreds of recognized subtypes based on different characteristics. The "O" antigen types and the "H" antigen types (also used in the subtyping of other bacteria) yield subtypes using differences in molecules on the surface of the bacteria. The designation of the most widely recognized subtype, *E. coli* O157:H7, relies on differences in both of these subtyping systems (Identified as #157 in the growing list of 181 different "O" antigens and #7 in the list of 53 "H" antigens). *E. coli* is probably the most thoroughly researched bacterial species, some of the

research having been prompted by the bacteria's important role in digestion. Other researchers are prompted by the rare but important subtypes associated with illnesses. Even within the studies on those subtypes that can cause disease, there are different category schemes. Illness results from a number of different and often sequential behaviors, and this has led to some commonly used ways to distinguish categories of *E. coli.*

Categories of those subtypes virulent in humans: Virulence factors
At least 3 virulence factors are commonly recognized: A factor that damages lining cells (intestine, other organs, and blood vessels); a factor that damages red blood cells (hemolysis); and toxins (resembling the shigatoxins produced by the bacteria Shigella dysenteriae). [1]

Many of the human illnesses are the result of bacterial toxin production. Subtypes that produce this toxin are collectively referred to as: Shiga Toxin *E. coli* (STEC). There are hundreds of subtypes of STEC, only a few of which have been associated with human illness. The equally small numbers of isolates that are shed from cows are mostly different from those found in humans. [2]

Another commonly used way of categorizing the virulent subtypes of *E. coli* is based on the nature of the disease they produce. The FDA's Bad Bug Book separates the virulent subtypes into four principal categories, based on the nature of the injury accompanying infection.

Categories of Principal Virulent Subtypes

1. Enterohemorrhagic (EHEC). [Hemorrhagic Colitis] These are the most well-known of the categories of current significance in public health. They are characterized by the breakup of red blood cells when there is infection. The *E. coli* O157:H7 subtype belongs in this category.

2. Enteropathogenic (EPEC). [Most common infantile diarrhea] This category causes watery diarrhea but the *E. coli* in this category do not produce any of the typical toxins seen in the other categories.

3. Enteroinvasive (EIEC). [Often referred to as bacillary dysentery] This category causes a mild form of dysentery.

4. Enterotoxigenic (ETEC). [Gastroenteritis or traveler's diarrhea] This category produces a mild form of illness with watery diarrhea. Worldwide, "traveler's diarrhea" is caused by this category and produces toxins related to a different bacterial genus, Shigella. However, destruction of red blood cells is not prominent.

With the current widespread public awareness of foodborne illnesses from the specific subtype *E. coli* O157:H7, tests were developed to easily identify this subtype in clinical laboratories. Unlike most forms of *E. coli*, this subtype was not able to utilize sorbitol as an energy source in laboratory cultures. Widely available and FDA-approved, procedures for distinguishing the O157:H7 subtype using antibody mixtures enables confirmation quickly and inexpensively. One of the consequences of the ready availability of the tests for the specific subtype O157:H7 is that other categories and subtypes causing diarrheal illness are not being recognized by hospital laboratories.

The enteropathogenic (EPEC) category of *E. coli* was once prominent in childhood diarrheal illness. During the 1960s and 70s, however, illness from this category became uncommon in the U.S. [3] This may be the result of acquired public immunity.

Disease Description

Animals

E. coli rarely causes illness in wild or domestic animals. However, subtypes that cause illness in humans may reside as temporary intestinal colonizers in domestic animals. It is commonly accepted that cattle feces are a major reservoir of *E. coli* O157:H7 in the U.S.

Humans

Acute, usually self-limiting gastroenteritis. The interval from consumption to symptoms is shorter than other foodborne enteritis, usually only a couple of days. Reviews show 100,000 illness, 3,000 hospitalizations, and 90 deaths annually in the U.S. from the subtypes with shigatoxins (STEC). [4] The frequency of different *E. coli* serotypes isolated from humans with illness varies significantly in different regions of the world.

Because there are multiple virulence factors, research discloses a considerable variety of strains with variation in human virulence and severity of illness. [5] The variation in the incidence of hemolytic uremic syndrome (HUS) in infants in different outbreaks is, in part, related to different forms of virulence factors and the types of shigatoxins produced by the specific subtype causing the diarrhea.

The prevalence of *E. coli* O157:H7 has been extensively studied. Human illnesses and cow colonization increase during warm months. Prevalence of colonization and shedding is higher in calves than in adult cows. Changes in feed causes changed prevalence in cows.

The normal intestinal microflora contains about 1,000,000,000 bacteria per gram of feces. Of these, as many as 1,000,000 colony forming units (cfu) are beneficial *E. coli*. Cows with transient colonization with *E. coli* O157:H7 usually shed about 500 cfu per gram of feces. There are reports of "supershedders" that may be more persistently colonized and shed higher numbers of organisms.

Report of Michigan Fresh Unprocessed Whole Milk Workgroup

SIDEBAR on Lateral Transfer of Genetic Material. [6]

Bacterial DNA has been studied extensively, and the DNA of *E. coli* more than any other bacteria. Of interest is the finding that the DNA that codes for several of the virulence factors, including the shigatoxins, originates from "lateral transfer" from other bacterial species. This is extremely complex and technical. However, understanding the basics of this process is critical to the understanding of virulence and the apparent disconnect between the naming of subtypes of *E. coli* and their ability to cause illness in humans.

Bacteriophages are viruses that infect bacteria. Typically, a specific bacteriophage is able to infect bacteria by attaching to its cell wall, inserting its genetic material into the cell, and subverting the normal activities of the bacteria into production of replicas of the bacteriophage's genetic material. It manufactures the structural components of the virus, assembles many new copies of the bacteriophage, disrupts/kills the infected bacterium, and disperses huge numbers of the bacteriophage.

On rare occasions when copies of the bacteriophage genetic material is being produced within an infected bacteria, random pieces of that bacteria's DNA can become inserted into the newly produced bacteriophage's genetic material. And on rare occasions when bacteriophage infect a bacterium, the process to make new bacteriophages aborts and the infected bacterium is not killed; instead, the injected genetic material remains and continues to be copied as that bacterium multiplies. So on extremely rare occasions, the ability to make new specific proteins is added to a bacterium's repertoire. And, on rare occasions, that "enhanced" bacteria is able to produce new protein that was not produced by its ancestors. All of these individual occasions are rare, but due to the huge number of times these things happen in the real world, remarkably unusual things do happen.

The shiga toxin in *E. coli* O157:H7 is similar to a toxin produced by the bacteria Shigella dysenteriae (responsible for endemic dysentery in many countries) and there is evidence that the appearance of the genetic code for this toxin present in uncommon subtypes of *E. coli* is an example of lateral transfer, via bacteriophage.

The more general "O" and "H" subtyping schemes are not based on the ability to cause illness. They are convenient and widely used when describing the *E. coli* subtypes, resulting in the important fact that simply because the subtype is E. coli O157:H7 does not categorize the subtype as one that causes disease in humans. There are people ill from *E. coli* infections, which have a subtype that is not O157:H7. Furthermore, not all *E. coli* O157:H7 are able to infect humans and cause illness.

Report of Michigan Fresh Unprocessed Whole Milk Workgroup

Category of Pathogen

The rare virulent forms of *E. coli* generally cause self-limiting acute enteritis with nausea, abdominal cramps, and mild diarrhea that can be bloody. The severity and pattern of symptoms varies considerably with various categories of virulent forms. As the general public is exposed to specific subtypes, immunity is acquired and the illness pattern shifts to other subtypes. The usual route of infection is oral, following consumption of food/drink or hand-to-mouth transfer.

SIDEBAR on Differing Perspectives.

Some of the confusion caused by the complexity of the different forms of *E. coli* is the result of the focus of different groups/laboratories that deal with these bacteria.

1. Research microbiologists see the full complexity of the forms of *E. coli*. They look for ways to organize that complexity into manageable categories, and develop methods that distinguish the forms that are the focus of their interest. The result is a proliferation of different methods to distinguish forms that behave in different ways.

2. The medical community and medical laboratories see *E. coli* as the cause of illness, and focus on diagnosing and treating the illnesses. They utilize rapid and convenient ways to determine the cause of diarrhea, and enable treatment as quickly as possible. The laboratories are equipped with the latest practical methods for detecting the current medically important subtypes. In practice all the isolates they encounter are virulent, having been obtained from people with significant diarrhea. There is no need to spend days and dollars to determine which category of disease since the patient's symptoms are indicators.

3. The agricultural school's interest in *E. coli* generally focuses on risk management. Attention is on detection, prevalence, and survival of forms of *E. coli*. They need techniques that are able to find the extremely uncommon forms identified as pathogens, within a world crowded with the generic forms.

The public health/epidemiology groups focus on surveillance and causation. They are interested in proving that isolates from a cluster of illnesses can be found in food/food establishments, and determining as convincingly as possible the source/cause of the illnesses so that they can prevent additional illness. They are interested in subtyping to the extent that it narrows the search, but rely on DNA techniques to enable matching. Serotyping is often predetermined by the submitting medical laboratories that rely on protocols that detect *E. coli* O157 when bloody stool is submitted from a child.

Report of Michigan Fresh Unprocessed Whole Milk Workgroup

Infectious dose
With the numerous subtypes and virulence forms it is difficult to give a specific infectious dose for the group. Reports range from 10 organisms to 100,000,000 organisms.

Complications of human infection
The most significant complication is hemolytic uremic syndrome (HUS). This complication has been studied extensively and has received considerable public attention. The true incidence is unknown but in the subset of hospitalized infants with bloody diarrhea caused by *E. coli* O157:H7, about 15% develop some degree of HUS. The syndrome includes damage to red blood cells and associated renal damage that can result in renal failure. [6]

Reservoirs

Water
Water does not naturally contain *E. coli*. However, water contaminated with *E. coli* from animal (including human) sources is very common.

Cattle
Cattle can become temporarily colonized by forms that are virulent in humans. These colonies shed in low numbers intermixed with the normal *E. coli* in the feces. Contaminated feed, drinking water, and contact with other cattle shedding the virulent forms of bacteria are significant sources of recolonization within the herd.

Humans
Humans are the ultimate source of human virulent forms of *E. coli*.

Other foods implicated in outbreaks
Ground beef is the most frequently implicated food source (USDA FSIA 5/10). Other foods include: leafy greens, seed sprouts, unbaked cookie dough, nuts, and fresh fruit juices.

Outbreaks for *E. coli* O157:H7
- Fresh unprocessed whole milk in Michigan 1999-2011 [7] – 0 illnesses

- Fresh unprocessed whole milk U.S. 1999-2011 [7] – Total 50 illnesses (average 4.6 per year)

- For all foods, estimated annual illnesses from E. coli O157:H7 in the U.S. based on data collected in 2006-2008 [8] – 63,153.

Report of Michigan Fresh Unprocessed Whole Milk Workgroup

General References

FDA "Bad Bug Book" Foodborne Pathogenic Microorganisms and Natural Toxins Handbook. [Cited url: www.cfsan.fda.gov/-mow/chapI.html Revised url: https://www.fda.gov/food/foodborne-pathogens/bad-bug-book-second-edition]

Note: the FDA Bad Bug Book includes different sections based on the category of *E. coli* categories rather than as a unified chapter.

Bach, et al. Transmission and control of Escherichia coli O157:H7 - A review. Can. J. of Anim. Sci., 82:475-490, 2002

Numbered Specific References

[1] CDC, Recommendations for diagnosis of shiga toxin--producing Escherichia coli infections by clinical laboratories, MMWR Oct, 16, 2009 58(RR12);1-14 [Cited url: www.cdc.gov/mmwr/preview/mmwrhtml/rr5812al.htm?s _cid=rr5812al _x _ Revised url: https://www.cdc.gov/mmwr/pdf/rr/rr5812.pdf]

[2] Baker, et al. 2007. Differences in Virulence among Escherichia coli O157:H7 Strains Isolated from Humans during Disease Outbreaks and from Healthy Cattle., Applied and Environmental Microbiology, 73 (22):7338-7346. http://aem.asm.org/cgi/content/short/73/22/7338

[3] Crane. 2010 Lessons from Enteropathogenic Escherichia coli. [Cited url, no longer available: www.microbemagazine.org/index.php?view=article&catid=365%3Afeatured&id=1410%3Alessons-from-enteropathogenic-escherichia-coli&tmpl=component&print=l&layout=default&page=&option=com_content&Itemid=437]

[4] Gould et al. 2009 MMWR Oct. 16, 2009/58:1-14. [Cited url: www.cdc.gov/mmwr/preview/mmwrhtml/rr5812al.htm Revised url: https://pubmed.ncbi.nlm.nih.gov/19834454/]

[5] Manning et al. 2008. Variation in virulence among clades of Escherichia coli O157:H7 associated with disease outbreaks. Proceedings of the National Academy of Science. www.pnas.org/cgi/doi/10.1073/pnas.0710834105

[6] Desch and Motto, 2007. Is There a Shared Pathophysiology for Thrombotic Thrombocytopenia Purpura and Hemolytic-Uremic-Syndrome? J. Am Soc. Nephrology 18:2475-2460.

[7] Illnesses enumerated for outbreaks were obtained from a comprehensive listing of incidents with official reports for the period, January 1, 1999 to March 30, 2011. All incidents were entered into the database from news releases and public reports

from national and state agencies, media articles, published listings from public interest groups, litigation websites and scientific publications, as well as from personal information. Numbers displayed in the Pathogen Summary documents include both confirmed and presumed illnesses given in final reports, without any evaluation of the way the officials made their determination. There is no judgment on the manner of the investigation nor on the strength of the conclusions. Only incidents within the U.S. were included, and only when the investigation specified consumption of fluid fresh unprocessed milk as the presumed source. Both cow and goat dairies that were specifically operated for the purpose of supplying fresh unprocessed milk to consumers were included.

[8] Foodborne Illness Acquired in the United States—Major Pathogens, Elaine Scallan, R.M. Hoekstra, F.J. Angulo, R.V. Tauxe, M.A. Widdowson, S.L. Roy, J.L. Jones and P.M. Griffin, Emerg. Infect. Dis. 2011. Table 2, pg. 16. Note that the numbers are specific for domestically acquired illnesses.

Scenarios for Transmission

> Throughout this section, items identified in **BOLD** are factors with the greatest potential for leading to illness.

Scenario(s) for Transmission of Virulent *Campylobacter jejuni* to People

Key requirements for transmission
- Must be virulent form of *C. jejuni*.
- Must be in adequate numbers (500 or more bacteria)
- Person must be susceptible (does not have full immunity), but not immunocompromised
- Must get into the intestinal tract of person (ingestion)

It's all about numbers. Microbiologists have worked hard to develop techniques/ conditions that enable jejuni to multiply in large numbers in the laboratory. However, in nature *C. jejuni* does not multiply outside of living cells of the animal intestine. During infection, virulent forms will multiply in the intestine. However, the principle of infectious dose is based on the observation that there must be a large enough mass of healthy virulent bacteria before infection happens. Becoming ill requires ingestion of adequate numbers of virulent *C. jejuni*. As a result, nearly all circumstances of foodborne *C. jejuni* illness involve contamination with large numbers so that enough survive the interval and conditions prior to ingestion.

Source and/or Vehicle for Transmission

People
- **People ill with diarrhea – the bacteria multiply and shed very high numbers of virulent *C. jejuni* in stool. Shedding persists after illness/ diarrhea has subsided. These subtypes are by nature virulent.**
- A carrier state with persistent high shedding is not well documented for *C. jejuni*.
- People with colonization that might transiently shed at low levels have not been described.
- People can be a vehicle for transmission of infectious stool to:
  - Other people
  - Animals
  - The environment, including water, feed, milk

Report of Michigan Fresh Unprocessed Whole Milk Workgroup

Animals
- **Poultry**
  - **Extremely high prevalence of *C. jejuni* in the intestine without causing illness. The bacteria multiply in the intestine and shed in high numbers within feces. There is a significant likelihood that the subtypes present would be virulent in humans.**
  - **Most likely to be the source of contamination from raw meat and juices during evisceration and processing in home and commercial food preparation areas.**
  - **Greatest risk of infection is from direct (physical) contact with living poultry.**

- **Cattle/cows**
  - Feces/manure
  - Cows can be colonized with limited multiplication of the bacteria and low shedding. These instances are transient and have variable subtypes over time and within a herd. These subtypes are unlikely to be virulent in humans.
  - Super-shedding has been documented. Multiplication is still limited but there can be persistent shedding. There is usually a persistent subtype in these instances, still unlikely to be virulent in humans.
  - Direct physical contact with manure on animals or on the ground.

Environment
- Feces – only significant if it contains high numbers of virulent bacteria
- Water – (must be contaminated with fecal material with high numbers of virulent bacteria). Survival is dependent on temperature and time.
- Biofilm – longer survival of *C. jejuni* within pre-formed biofilm from non-pathogen bacteria (*C. jejuni* are motile)
  - **Persistent within equipment, piping, containers, under normal cleaning operations (experts consider this the most significant source of contamination of milk).**
  - Requires mechanical scrubbing to remove from surfaces
  - **Microscopic flakes of biofilm carry embedded bacteria and are not easily diluted, resulting in uneven distribution.**
- Animal Feed (contaminated with feces/manure)
  - Shared feeding; not significant since would need bacteria in the mouth
  - Distributed on the ground where there is feces/manure
  - Secondarily contaminated with contaminated water
  - Contaminated by person shedding high numbers

Milk
- It may be theoretically possible with *C. jejuni* mastitis to shed directly into milk from the udder, but may only have been reported once in the literature
- Contamination of milk after milking

Report of Michigan Fresh Unprocessed Whole Milk Workgroup

- From any of the previously listed sources but must be in high concentration
- Should be visible in a milk filter if contamination is manure. (Milk filters are designed to trap large particles and make such contamination more conspicuous)
- Incidental contamination would usually be diluted in the bulk tank.
- There is poor survival in fresh whole milk at refrigerated temperatures.
- Combination of factors that inhibit multiplication of bacteria in fresh milk (see Topic 2 – Benefits and Values). A decrease in numbers of any bacteria in milk reduces the effectiveness of these inhibitions.
- Rinse water contaminated with milk (increased survival)
- **Microscopic flakes of biofilm in bulk tank, milk lines, milking equipment (not visible). Might pass through milk filter.**

Other foods
- **Fresh poultry meat**
- Fresh shellfish (rarely *C. jejuni*)
- Leafy vegetables (biofilm) contaminated by bird feces containing virulent forms of *C. jejuni*.
- **Any food contaminated by a person shedding high numbers of virulent forms**

Contamination of containers by people, contaminated water, fecal/manure
- Food containers – inside or outside
- Transportation containers or equipment.

Scenario(s) for Transmission of Virulent
Listeria monocytogenes to People

- Must be virulent form of *L. monocytogenes*

- Virulent form must be in adequate numbers to cause illness

- Assumes person must be susceptible (does not have full immunity)

- Generally, assumes transmission by ingestion

Most cases of human listeriosis are not associated with investigated outbreaks. Since the sporadic cases are rarely investigated, there is little information on the modes of transmission or sources of the virulent form of *L. monocytogenes*. This is further complicated due to the potential of long incubation times. Conclusions on definitive sources, reservoirs, and modes of transmission are also distorted since outbreaks from *L. monocytogenes* are extremely rare and vary considerably.

The systemic form of human "foodborne listeriosis is a relatively rare but serious disease with high fatality rates (20%-30%) compared to other foodborne microbial pathogens." [1]

Being elderly or a child is not in itself a major risk factor for listeriosis. However, conditions that are more likely to occur in different age groups (leukemia, cancer, dialysis, use of immunosuppressive drugs) are major risk factors.

Nearly all cases of foodborne listeriosis in humans are associated with consumption of very high numbers of virulent organisms, and are associated with foods and food handling that enable multiplication of the bacteria prior to consumption.

It is generally accepted that the general public consumes food contaminated with *L. monocytogenes*, occasionally and repeatedly, throughout their lives. There is little information on the immunological effect of this exposure.

Source and/or Vehicle for Transmission
People
- People with gastrointestinal illness – during these illnesses the bacteria multiply and shed in very high numbers of the causative subtype of *L. monocytogenes* in their stool.
- Adults with systemic infections (listeriosis) have organisms in their blood stream as well as very high concentrations of *L. monocytogenes* within the infected organs. Other people are unlikely to become infected from contact with the ill person.
- A carrier state with persistent high shedding is not well documented for *L. monocytogenes*.

Report of Michigan Fresh Unprocessed Whole Milk Workgroup

- People with colonization that might transiently shed at low levels are most common within populations that have greater exposure to environmental *L. monocytogenes*, such as farmers and meat processors. Recent studies show a small number of the general adult public may intermittently shed *L. monocytogenes* in their stool without symptoms, but it is not known if these were virulent forms.
- People could be a vehicle for transmission of infectious bacteria in their stool to:
  - Other people. People exposed to cases of listeriosis may transiently shed *L. monocytogenes* in their stool, but rarely have symptoms
  - Animals
  - The environment, including water and feed

Current reviews conclude that the findings listed above are not significant contributors to human illnesses.

In contrast, pregnant women with *L. monocytogenes* in their blood stream, even if not significantly ill themselves, are the principal source of transmission to their fetus or newborn.

Animals
- Cattle/cows, sheep, and goats
  - Feces/manure
    - Cows can be colonized with limited multiplication of the bacteria and low shedding in manure. These instances are transient, have variable subtypes over time and within a herd, and the subtypes are unlikely to be virulent in humans.
    - Super-shedding is reported. Multiplication is still limited but there can be persistent shedding. These may be a significant contributor to herd exposure; however, the subtypes are unlikely to be virulent in humans.
- **Infected fetuses, newborns, and products of conception (amniotic fluid, placenta, and blood) contain large numbers of forms virulent in the animals. Workers exposed to these materials may become infected. These materials also contribute to the cycling of *L. monocytogenes* in the general farm environment.**
- Wild, land, and aquatic animals are not considered a significant source for human listeriosis.

Environment
- *L. monocytogenes* is widely distributed in the environment.
- **Silage – Poorly managed silage is generally accepted as the principal source of listeriosis in cows/cattle. A greater variety of strains are isolated from silage than from animal infections, suggesting that far**

Report of Michigan Fresh Unprocessed Whole Milk Workgroup

more strains will multiply in poorly managed silage than are able to cause infection in exposed domestic animals.

- Feces – Generally accepted as a source of *L. monocytogenes* in the farm environment. However, there are far more strains of *L. monocytogenes* in the environment than in the farm's animals. Manure spread on fields may contribute to contaminated crops. This has been shown to be a source of human listeriosis, particularly when the crop was subsequently stored in cool, damp conditions for months (e.g. cabbage). Fecal contamination of foods entering processing plants may contribute to the introduction of *L. monocytogenes* into processing plant environments.
- Water contamination is a significant source, present in reservoirs and as a transmitter of environmental listeria. It is a component of the generalized contamination in the farm environment
- Animal Feed other than silage may be contaminated with feces/manure or water.
- Can be contaminated by person shedding high numbers.

Current reviews conclude that the sources listed above are not significant as the source or transmission resulting in human listeriosis.

More Significant Sources or Methods of Transmission of *L. monocytogenes* to Humans

- Biofilm – There is longer survival of *L. monocytogenes* within biofilm. Although the ability to form their own biofilm is variable among different strains, given time, strains with poor production of biofilm are able to establish biofilm.
  - **Biofilm is important to the persistence within the processing plant environment, equipment, piping and containers, under normal cleaning operations.**
  - Requires physical cleansing to remove from surfaces.
- **Microscopic fragments of biofilm carry embedded bacteria. Such fragments do not easily dilute in the product, resulting in uneven distribution.**
- **Processing environments: Commercial, retail, and home food processing environments are considered the most significant contributor to human listeriosis. These locations and handling practices harbor and enhance the ability of *L. monocytogenes* to multiply slowly and persistently over extremely long periods; they compete in the environmental ecosystems at refrigerated temperatures and contaminate a variety of foods. Slicing of processed refrigerated meats is one of the riskiest procedures.**
- **Contaminated water is a significant source, both in the reservoir and as a transmitter of environmental listeria in processing plants.**

Report of Michigan Fresh Unprocessed Whole Milk Workgroup

Milk
- Mastitis is an uncommon location for systemic listeriosis in cows, but might contribute to spread in a herd. However, the pattern of strains virulent in cows is different to that of clinical cases in humans.
- Contamination of milk after milking:
  - Contamination from manure would require a very large amount to reach infectious doses.
  - Contamination from other dairy environmental sources, with conditions that enable multiplication of *L. monocytogenes*, including drains and residual wash water.
  - There is poor survival of inoculated *L. monocytogenes* in fresh whole milk, even at refrigerated temperatures.
- Processed milk has been linked to rare outbreaks of listeriosis. However, this contamination was from the processing environment and not from inadequate pasteurization or from contamination with pre-pasteurized milk. *L. monocytogenes* is capable of multiplication in processed milk. Most problems with dairy products have been related to cheese.
- Although fresh unprocessed whole milk would qualify as a ready-to-eat food, unprocessed fluid milk does not fit the conclusion that ready-to-eat foods are a significant source of listeriosis. This is due to the fact that the most significant risk is in the processing of the foods.

Fresh unprocessed whole milk has not been linked to human cases of listeriosis in the U.S. over the last 10 years.

Other foods
- **All reviews and risk analyses conclude that processed foods (ready-to-eat foods) are the principal source of all of the types of foodborne listeriosis. The patterns in these outbreaks implicate the processing plants themselves and not the specific food. Environmental contamination in food processing operations with *L. monocytogenes* is widespread and persistent. Risk factors include: the plants themselves, the equipment, packaging, and storage. Risk significantly increases with the length of storage under refrigeration of the processed product. Recently it has been shown that food delivery services such as deli-type establishments appear to increase the risk for processed meats that are served cold.**

- Intact, fresh, unprocessed, or undamaged foods have not been linked to human listeriosis.

References

FDA Bad Bug Book. Listeria, listeriosis, and food safety, Third Edition. 2007 Ryser and Marth.

Numbered Specific References

[1] Risk assessment of Listeria monocytogenes in ready-to-eat foods. WHO, FAQ 2004

Scenario(s) for Transmission of Virulent Salmonella spp. to People

* Must be a salmonella subtype virulent in people
* Virulent form must be in adequate numbers to cause illness
* Applied to the general population (do not have full immunity or compromised immune condition)
* Generally, assumes transmission by ingestion

The vast majority of cases of human salmonellosis are not associated with investigated outbreaks. Since the sporadic cases are rarely investigated, there is little information on the sources or modes of transmission of the virulent subtypes of Salmonella spp. Conclusions on definitive sources, reservoirs, and modes of transmission are also distorted since outbreaks from Salmonella spp. are extremely rare, the subtypes are usually different, and outbreak characteristics vary considerably. When outbreaks are recognized, they often include large numbers of illnesses, significant rates of hospitalization, and some deaths. Systemic infections are uncommon. However, in very rare large outbreaks, the pattern suggests a more virulent form, with more systemic infections (predominately in the elderly with associated debilitating conditions) associated with increased rates of hospitalization and more deaths.

Because typhoid fever (caused by the subtype *Salmonella enterica* serovar Typhi) is not a significant health problem in the U.S. at this time, it is not included in this summary.

Nearly all cases of foodborne salmonellosis in people are associated with consumption of high numbers of virulent organisms, and are associated with foods and food handling that enable multiplication of the bacteria prior to consumption.

It is generally accepted that the general public, occasionally and repeatedly, consumes food contaminated with various subtypes of salmonella throughout their lives. There is little information on the immunological effect of this exposure.

There have been a number of studies that looked at human cases. Each tends to have their own pattern of virulent subtypes and sources. These change with time, region, and method of collecting isolates. It is common to find studies that span longer periods of time and show changes in prevalence (both increases and declines) over years. This may be the result of changes in public immunity levels, or alterations in the expression of virulent factors in the subtypes.

Source and/or Vehicle for Transmission

People
- With gastrointestinal illness – During these illnesses the bacteria multiply and are shed with very high numbers of salmonella in the stool.
- Excluding typhoid fever, a carrier state with persistent high shedding is not well documented for the subtypes of salmonella virulent in humans.
- People could be a vehicle for transmission of infectious bacteria in their stool to:
  o Other people through handling of food.
  o The environment, including water and feed.

Animals
- All domestic animals have significant disease caused by Salmonella spp. However, the specific subtypes are frequently animal specific.
- Human illness results from consumption of meat or meat products that have been processed, stored, or served under conditions that enable multiplication of salmonella.
- **Eggs can be contaminated on the outside from poultry shedding salmonella**
- **Egg content can be infected with the *Salmonella enterica Enteritidis* from hens with ovarian infections.**
- Wild, land, and aquatic animals also have significant disease but the subtypes are frequently animal specific. **Human illness associated with animal disease usually results from direct physical contact with a pet that is sick or shedding high numbers of a virulent subtype.**
- **A carrier state within animal groups is well recognized as a source of transmission to humans through: direct contact, ingestion of meat, or from contamination of other food products.**

Environment
- Water contamination is a significant source, both reservoir and transmitter of environmental salmonella, and is a component of the generalized contamination in the farm environment. **It is also a significant source of transmission to humans.**
- Animal Feeds may be contaminated through direct contact with animals or humans, feces/manure, or water.
- **Processing environments: Many of the recent outbreaks have been traced to processed foods, where the processing environment has been contaminated. However, trace backs have also implicated specific ingredients (that both directly introduce virulent bacteria, or**

Report of Michigan Fresh Unprocessed Whole Milk Workgroup

contaminate the processing environment/equipment). Ingredients are often processed, and the processing environment or the source of the ingredient may have contributed to the spread.

Milk
- Mastitis is an uncommon location for salmonella infection in cows. The subtypes virulent in cows are different from the subtypes associated with human illnesses.
  - Contamination of milk after milking
  - Contamination from manure would require very large amounts of contaminant to reach infectious doses in the farm tank
  - Contamination from other dairy environmental sources. This would be significant only with conditions that enable multiplication of Salmonella, such as in animal feed
  - There is poor survival of inoculated Salmonella spp. in fresh whole milk at refrigerated temperatures

Other foods
- Although many foods have been associated with human salmonella gastroenteritis, with the exception of eggs, there is no real pattern for specific foods. Almost every cluster of illness is associated with a different food. Current outbreaks, although rare, can be large and each are associated with contamination of a specific food. However, most have in common handling, storage, or serving conditions that enable multiplication of salmonella.
- **In contrast, the outbreaks caused by *Salmonella enterica Enteritidis* are specifically caused by eggs infected within the laying hens.**
-

Major Reference

FDA Bad Bug Book (distribute 2010 article from MSU on Michigan farm with salmonella)

Scenario(s) for Transmission of Virulent *E. coli* to People

- Must be a virulent form of *E. coli*

- The subtype O157:H7 has the most abundant and reliable information; therefore the scenario will focus on this subtype (serotype)

- Must be in adequate numbers (10 or more bacteria in serving consumed)

- Person must be susceptible (does not have full immunity, but is not immunocompromised)

- Must enter the intestinal tract of person (ingestion) to cause illness

Infection and Illness

There has been discussion about the distinction between infection (meaning establishment of bacteria with multiplication in, or on, the cells of the intestine) and illness (meaning persons with symptoms such as diarrhea, abdominal pain, fever, etc.) This distinction is not always important in understanding epidemiology of foodborne illnesses, however, with the virulent forms of *E. coli* there is some advantage to understanding this. Obviously, illness does not happen without infection. But infection does not automatically mean illness. With certain bacteria, persistent infection in the absence of illness is described as a carrier state. In the case of the virulent forms of *E. coli*, a true carrier state has not been reported. However, a transient colonization with modest multiplication, either prior to the onset of symptoms or without symptoms, is possible in humans and is the dominant situation in cattle *(e.g., E. coli* O157:H7).

It's all about numbers

Suitable conditions for *E. coli* multiplication are widespread, primarily within the intestines of most animals, but also many foods (intact, damaged, processed, or cooked). During human illnesses, virulent forms will multiply in the intestine and shed large numbers in the diarrheic stool. Becoming ill requires ingestion of adequate numbers of virulent *E. coli*, however with the O157:H7 subtype, the commonly accepted infectious dose is 10 bacteria in a serving. Some human studies cite higher numbers for infectious dose, and with other serotypes the accepted dose is much higher. Much of the epidemiological information about human illness with the virulent strains of *E. coli* O157:H7 is more easily understood if you consider that there is an initial stage of infection, with illness following in some of the infected people.

Although there are abundant conditions favorable for the multiplication of the common *E. coli*, large numbers of studies using *E. coli* O157:H7 establish that, with this subtype, there is a reduction in numbers over time, rather than multiplication. Survival is the consistent measurement, not multiplication.

Report of Michigan Fresh Unprocessed Whole Milk Workgroup

Except for active infectious disease when the virulent forms are present from contamination of feces, the non-virulent forms are present in far greater numbers, and competitively multiply more rapidly than the virulent forms. There is a study that showed increases in *E. coli* O157:H7 when inoculated into mismanaged silage, and some reports of increases in the intestinal tract of common flies and birds when allowed to ingest contaminated material.

Source and/or Vehicle for Transmission (subtype O157:H7)

People
- **People ill with diarrhea—the virulent forms, including the subtype O157:H7, multiply and shed in very high numbers and are the dominant bacteria in their stool. Shedding persists after illness/ diarrhea has subsided. The subtypes that are shed with diarrhea are, by nature, virulent.**
- A carrier state with persistent high shedding is not well documented for *E. coli* O157:H7.
- People with colonization that might transiently shed at low levels have not been described in the literature.
- **People can be a vehicle for transmission of infectious stool to:**
  - **Other people. Data from outbreak investigations consistently document secondary illness in people in physical contact with those with illness.** The percentage of the cases that are considered to be secondary infections is not large. However, the data may be skewed since it is possible that many of the contacts do not become primarily ill because they have some degree of prior immunity. Given that likelihood, the percentage of secondary infections may be underestimated due to that same prior immunity. In an epidemiological analysis by the CDC of U.S. outbreaks from 1982-2002, published in 2005 by Rangel, et al., 21 percent were associated with ground beef, 21 percent unknown, and the next highest was person-to-person which was 14 percent. All dairy products were 2 percent.
  - Animals – see below.
- **The environment, including water, feed, milk, containers, food preparation surfaces, and food.**

Animals
- Cattle/cows – High prevalence of *E. coli* O157:H7 in the intestine without causing illness. The bacteria colonize the intestine (highest rate in the end of the colon) and shed in low numbers within feces (500 cfu/gram of feces). Colonization is more frequent in calves and heifers. There are occasional **"super-shedders", which shed at higher numbers (-1,000 cfu/gram feces) and persist with a single strain of *E. coli* O157:H7**
- Other animals

Report of Michigan Fresh Unprocessed Whole Milk Workgroup

- Feces/manure from domestic animals
  - o Can be colonized with limited multiplication of the bacteria and low shedding. These instances are transient, and have variable subtypes over time and within a herd; subtypes are unlikely to be virulent in humans.
  - o Super-shedding is reported. Multiplication is still limited but there can be persistent shedding. Fecal contamination (other than from human diarrhea) will contain all other fecal bacteria in their normal relative numbers. Therefore, any virulent forms will be subject to the competitive inhibition and other factors that suppress multiplication. Furthermore, any food that is contaminated with fecal material will have extremely high levels of background fecal bacteria, intermixed with any rare *E. coli* O157:H7 that happens to be present.
- Direct physical contact with manure on animals or the ground.
- *E. coli* O157:H7 has been isolated from bird feces and flies.

Environment
(All are examples of contamination; note the source and studies document the rate of survival, not increase in numbers)
- Feces – only significant if it contains high enough numbers of virulent bacteria. Numbers decline with time.
- Water – (must be contaminated with fecal material with high numbers of virulent bacteria). Survival within contaminants is dependent on temperature and time.
- Biofilm – survival of *E. coli* O157:H7 within preformed biofilm. Preformed from non-pathogen bacteria or produced by *E. coli* O157:H7. Persistent within equipment, piping, and containers, under normal cleaning operations. Requires physical cleansing to remove from surfaces.
- Biofilm produced by *E. coli* O157:H7 is well studied. It forms within the intestinal contents but also on the lining cell surface of the colon.
- **Microscopic fragments of biofilm carrying embedded bacteria. These free-floating fragments do not easily distribute, resulting in uneven distribution.**

Animal Feed
When contaminated with feces/manure or by oral bacteria through shared feeding.
- Distributed on ground that has feces/manure on it
- Secondarily contaminated with contaminated water
- **Contaminated by person shedding high numbers**
- In cattle herds the intermittent recycling of strains of E. coli O157:H7 is likely to result from re-ingestion from contaminated feed, water, and other environmental contacts. However, there is no evidence that the total population of *E. coli* O157:H7 increases under these conditions. [see separate diagram of cycle that follows below]

Report of Michigan Fresh Unprocessed Whole Milk Workgroup

Milk
- As the direct/primary source. Theoretically it may be possible with *E. coli* mastitis shedding directly into milk from the udder.
- Contamination of milk during and after milking
  - From any of above sources, but must be in high concentration. Should be visible in the milk filter if contamination is manure. Milk filters are designed to trap large particles and make such contamination more conspicuous.
  - Incidental contamination would usually be diluted in the bulk tank.
  - There is poor survival in fresh whole milk at refrigerated temperatures (Massa et al. 1999). [1]
  - Combination of factors that inhibit multiplication of bacteria in fresh milk. (see Topic 2 – Benefits and Values)
- Rinse water contaminated with milk (increased survival compared to whole milk)
- **The microscopic fragments from biofilm in bulk tank, milk lines, and milking equipment**

Other foods
- **Ground beef**
- Leafy vegetables contaminated by manure, water, and human contact; **increases with damage, cutting, and plant diseases**
- **Fruit juices when fruit is contaminated (by humans, on the ground, by flies)**
- **Any food contaminated by person shedding high numbers of a virulent form.**

Contamination of containers by people, contaminated water, fecal/manure
- Bottle inside or on outside
- Transportation containers or equipment

Report of Michigan Fresh Unprocessed Whole Milk Workgroup

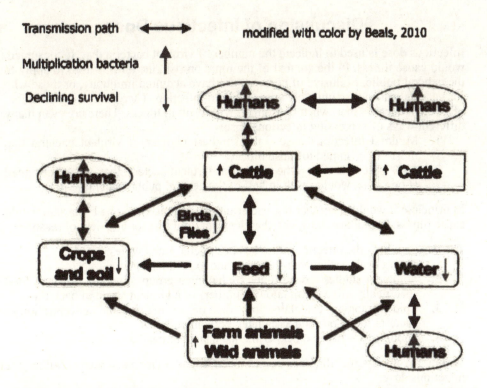

Fig. 1. Transmission of *E. coli* O157:H7 in the environment giving rise to a cycle of infection that may enable maintenance of the organism in cattle herds. Effective control of E. coli O1S7:H7 requires suppression at as many points in the cycle as possible, in order to minimize the incidence of foodborne disease associated with this human pathogen. Bach et al, 2002 [2]

Numbered Specific References

[1] Massa, S.E. et al 1999 Fate of Escherichia coli O157:H7 in unpasteurized milk stored at 8°C. Letters in Applied Microbiology 28(1):89-92.

[2] Bach, S.J. et al 2002. Transmission and control of Escherichia coli O157:H7 – A review. Can. J. Animal Sci. 82:475-490.

Discussion of Infectious Dose

Infectious dose is used to indicate the number of virulent bacteria that, if consumed, would cause illness. In the context of the topic on risk, the term is used to apply to the general public, exclusive of persons who have acquired immunity, or those who for various reasons are uniquely susceptible to infection. There is no single number of virulent bacteria that, when consumed, will result in illness. There are even many different ways of expressing infectious dose:

1. Minimal infectious dose – the smallest number of virulent bacteria that must be consumed to cause illness.
2. 50% infectious dose – the number of virulent bacteria that, when consumed at one time, would result in half of the general public becoming ill.

In principle it would seem that if a bacterium is virulent, even one bacterium would cause illness. In practice, however, that does not hold true for a variety of reasons.

The way in which the infectious dose has been determined varies:

1. Theoretical – calculated from real and experimental data
2. Volunteer studies – determined by having a group of people consume food specifically mixed with known numbers of a virulent strain of bacteria
3. Epidemiologic – calculated from data on serving size and concentration of bacteria found on food associated with an outbreak
4. Laboratory – based on experiments, using animals

Within the foodborne illnesses it has been found that many factors affect the infectious dose:

1. Virulence of the specific strain of bacteria
2. Nature of the food with which the bacteria are associated
3. Other food ingested at the same time
4. Serving size
5. Sequence of repetitive consumption of individual servings
6. Individual differences in personal susceptibility
7. Differences in the environment of the intestinal tract of the specific individual consuming the food
8. Health, concurrent medications, or concurrent illnesses of the person consuming the food
9. Health/vitality of the bacteria consumed

It is unusual to have the specific criteria used to define the infectious dose explained, when the term is generally used. Except in specific instances the number used in the Workgroup's Summary Statements is the "generally or widely accepted" number.

Report of Michigan Fresh Unprocessed Whole Milk Workgroup

Other Pathogens of Historical Milk-Related Public Health Concerns

In the late 1800s several epidemic diseases dominated the public health scene in the U.S. As advocates for laws requiring pasteurization organized their campaigns, they focused the public on the role of milk in several of these diseases. Although only one of these, human tuberculosis, continues to be a significant public health concern, each are reviewed here for historical value.

(See also Topic 1 – History)

Diphtheria is caused by the bacteria *Corynebacterium diphtheriae*, a virulent pathogen host adapted to humans. This is a severe infection of the upper respiratory area. *Corynebacterium diphtheriae* is essentially an obligate parasite of humans, transmitted between people. It is not a zoonotic disease (it does not grow in cows or other animals). Historically, examples of localized outbreaks of diphtheria were linked to persons with active infections or human carriers who were milking, processing, or distributing milk. The organism does not survive long in the environment, and does not grow in milk. Pasteurization does kill these bacteria in milk. Pasteurization would only be an effective form of protection in those extremely rare circumstances when large numbers of virulent bacteria contaminated the milk itself, from an infected person or carrier coughing directly into the milk, or from sputum containing large numbers of the virulent bacteria getting into the milk from handling prior to pasteurization. The majority of these clusters were linked to people handling the milk after pasteurization would have occurred, and during distribution to homes. Diphtheria was effectively controlled by public health interventions, specifically mandated immunization of the public. Examination of the medical records show that the number of cases had a uniform steady decline starting (1880s) well before pasteurization was commercially used, and had a very low incident at the time mandatory pasteurization was adopted in the U.S.

Scarlet fever is a group of skin disease that can include significant upper respiratory infection caused by forms of streptococci that produce a toxin that destroys red blood cells. Regional epidemics have occurred throughout the world, including significant occurrences at different times in the mid- to late-1800s and 1900s in the U.S. In the epidemic occurrences, the disease is highly contagious through person-to-person contact. A few investigations of localized clusters of scarlet fever in the early 1900s were attributed to milk handlers who had skin rashes. The real relevance of these cases was that they were published because of the distinct finding of a link between cause and effect. A consistent finding in these cases was that the infection originated from a milk handler (not the animals). In some of these historical reports, boiling the milk protected the family. The milkborne spread of the pathogen may have contributed in a minor way to the

Report of Michigan Fresh Unprocessed Whole Milk Workgroup

general public health impact of scarlet fever during this period in history. During the turn of the century (1890-1920) physicians were only beginning to associate skin rashes with scarlet fever. Milking was by hand and contamination of fresh milk from a rash on the hands was possible. However, the significant route of transmission of the epidemic forms was historically, and continues to be today, by direct physical contact between people. The significant public health impact of scarlet fever was nearly eliminated with the recognition that: the disease was caused by bacteria; skin rashes were associated with severe respiratory infection; people with the infection should be isolated and those with skin rashes should be kept from handling food, including milk.

Bovine tuberculosis is a chronic debilitating disease of cows caused by *Mycobacterium bovis*. The disease was endemic in the U.S. during the late 1800s and first half of the 1900s. Incidence in domestic herds in Michigan was above 30% in some areas. Severely infected cows can shed bacteria in their feces and, with active mastitis, directly into milk. The cows become ill over long periods of time and are extremely sick, and milk production drops significantly. Infection can be transmitted to other animals and, to a limited extent, to humans. Human infection is acquired predominately by direct physical contact with a severely ill animal. There is rare documentation of transmission to people from consuming heavily contaminated milk. Pasteurization is effective against this bacterium. Unlike human tuberculosis which is transmitted through airborne droplets, the bovine form does not spread through the air. When human infection of the bovine form is from consumption of milk or hand-to-mouth transfer, very large numbers of virulent organisms must be introduced. The disease is localized in the lymph nodes of the neck, or along the intestinal tract. During the late 1800s and early 1900s, it was difficult to distinguish the bovine disease from the human form and many scientists believed they were the same disease. However, now that we know that the human form is a disease of the lungs, and the bovine form is a disease of the regions of the intestinal tract from the mouth to the abdomen; the disease in humans can be distinguished and differentiated. The number of "extrapulmonary" forms in people was small compared to the pulmonary forms. Public health records of the time, which included the small number of bovine forms of disease, show a uniform steady decline starting well before pasteurization was commercially used, and with a very persistent low incidence at the time mandatory pasteurization was adopted in the U.S. Because the bovine disease had a significant economic impact on cattle and dairy operations, an aggressive federal eradication program of testing and killing has essentially eliminated the disease in the U.S. And an active surveillance program continues to watch for and eradicate the disease imported from other countries. Currently, Michigan has a specific problem due to persistent bovine tuberculosis in deer and other animals in a confined region of the Lower Peninsula, and is spending considerable resources to protect the domestic cattle herds from any chance of spread. Bovine tuberculosis is not a current public health risk in the U.S.

Report of Michigan Fresh Unprocessed Whole Milk Workgroup

Human tuberculosis is a disease caused by *Mycobacterium tuberculosis*. This form of tuberculosis is primarily a chronic disease of the lungs that may last for years without any symptoms, but can become active if the person's immune system is compromised. When the disease is active, and in rarer circumstances of dissemination throughout the body, these debilitated persons can infect other people. Infection is predominately spread through airborne droplets containing the virulent pathogen which, when inhaled, causes infection in the lungs. This organism is an intracellular obligate parasite in humans. In the vast majority of cases the organism grows slowly within cells of the lung, does not cause illness, and is not infectious. This is not a zoonotic disease, other animals do not become infected from humans, and spread does not occur from animals, including cows. Although bovine and human tuberculosis are fundamentally different diseases, during the late 1800s the distinction was not widely recognized. "Tuberculosis" was epidemic in the U.S. and a major public health concern. As a result, advocates of pasteurization were able to argue that "tuberculosis", that was known to be a disease of cows, was being transmitted from the cows through milk. The small proportion of "tuberculosis" in the bovine form is discussed above. The major proportion of "tuberculosis" that is human does not infect cows, and therefore cannot be transmitted through milk. There were people with tuberculosis that were milking, processing, and distributing milk. Milk and milk containers could only be a vehicle for transmission of human tuberculosis in the rare circumstance that the milkers or handlers had active tuberculosis and were coughing up infectious sputum. And although pasteurization was ultimately managed so that it would kill most *Mycobacterium tuberculosis*, pasteurization would only have intervened in the transmission from humans to humans, if the contamination from infected sputum occurred prior to when pasteurization would have occurred. If Mycobacterium tuberculosis was present in milk, it would cause disease of the intestinal lymph nodes (not the lungs) and only if present in extremely high numbers. Clinical studies have shown that nearly all intestinal tuberculosis is the result of a person with active human pulmonary disease swallowing sputum containing huge numbers of the pathogen. If transmission of human tuberculosis occurred in association with milk, it is far more likely that it would have been from contamination of the outside of milk bottles with drying and airborne distribution. Human tuberculosis was epidemic in the U.S. and persists as a small but significant public health problem today. Pasteurization of milk is unlikely to have ever been a significant intervention in the epidemic. Examination of the historical medical records show that the number of cases of "tuberculosis" had a uniform steady decline starting (1880s) well before pasteurization was commercially used, and with a very low incident at the time mandatory pasteurization was adopted in the U.S.

Typhoid fever is a human disease caused by *Salmonella enterica* subtype Typhi. This bacterium is an obligate parasite of humans. It is not a zoonotic disease and does not infect other animals. Typhoid fever was epidemic in the U.S. during the 1800s and early 1900s. It is transmitted from person to person through ingestion of material contaminated from the stools of infected people, or rare carriers, and from drinking contaminated water. Historically, examples of localized outbreaks of typhoid fever were linked to persons with active infections or human carriers who were milking, processing, or distributing milk. The advocates of mandatory pasteurization used these incidents in their campaigns. Pasteurization does kill these bacteria in milk. Pasteurization would only be protective in those extremely rare circumstances when large numbers of virulent bacteria from an infected person or from a carrier's feces was introduced directly into the milk from handling prior to pasteurization. The majority of those clusters investigated and published were linked to people handling the milk, after pasteurization would have occurred, and during distribution of milk to homes. Typhoid fever in the U.S. has been effectively controlled by public health interventions, including: public (both municipal and rural) water and sewage management; isolation and treatment of carriers; and human immunization. Examination of the historical medical records show that the number of deaths had a uniformly steady decline starting well before pasteurization was commercially used, and with a very low incident at the time mandatory pasteurization was adopted in the U.S.

Brucellosis (undulant fever, Bang's disease)

Brucellosis is a serious disease in many domestic animals, including cows, caused by members of the genus brucella. Each species of brucella tends to predominate in a group of animals and have different patterns of disease; however, crossover between animal groups can occur. The species associated with human disease is also variable. The natural environment for the growth and multiplication of these bacteria is inside the cells of animals. In humans, brucellosis can present with acute symptoms, but may also take months before symptoms become evident. Fever, with a characteristic undulating pattern, and generalized weakness are a manifestation of the systemic spread of the infection. Most human infections are the result of direct physical contact with infected animals, or material from infected animal abortions.

In cows, goats, and sheep there is a tendency for the disease to include infections of the mammary glands and the uterus. Milk production is significantly reduced in infected animals. Even so, infected dairy animals can shed large numbers of the bacteria in the milk they produce. The milk ring test has been historically available to quickly detect a cow with brucella mastitis. The current standards for pasteurization are set to inactivate brucella in milk. Historically, milkborne brucellosis in humans was a significant public health risk. Due to the economic impact of reduced milk production and reproductive failures, a nationally mandated program to eliminate brucellosis in cattle was initiated in the 1950s. This aggressive "test-and-kill the herd" policy has effectively eradicated the disease in cattle and cows. As a result, human brucellosis has become extremely rare in the U.S., and is found predominately in immigrants and foreign travelers.

Categories of Risk
Other Than Infectious Disease for People
Consuming Fresh Unprocessed Whole Milk

Allergies to milk
These are immunologic reactions in individuals to some components of milk, nearly all of which are triggered by proteins. These reactions are classified as hypersensitivity because they can be triggered by very small amounts of milk, or the presence of very small amounts of the specific allergic component in non-dairy products. It is generally accepted that the proteins that trigger these reactions must migrate from inside the intestine into the tissues and intercellular spaces of the body, intact (not digested), to initiate the reaction. Therefore "permeability" of the intestinal lining cells is an important factor in the initial sensitivity, and in the triggering of subsequent reactions. The severity of the reaction is different in different people, ranging from mild symptoms to sudden, life-threatening conditions with significant numbers of deaths. Milk allergies are considered the second most common food allergy after allergies to eggs. Because of the large number of people affected, the widespread use of milk or milk proteins in prepared foods, and the fact that the reactions are triggered by very small amounts, food labeling regulations require it to be stated if there are any milk protein ingredients in the product.

Early childhood cow's milk allergy
This allergy adversely affects 2%-8% of infants in the U.S. This is a reaction to cow's milk, usually seen once a newborn child is weaned from human breast milk to commercial formulas. Some studies show that the same reaction may occur with goat or sheep milk. The infant reacts with a variety of symptoms, including simple refusal to drink the formula, rashes (the most common reaction), vomiting, diarrhea, and, rarely, acute pulmonary distress. One of the characteristics of this immunologic reaction is that as the child grows older, the sensitivity to the protein allergen in the milk goes away within a few years.

Persistent casein milk allergy
It adversely affects 1%-4% of the adult public in the U.S. This allergy is well recognized, however the relationship with childhood cow's milk allergy is still being researched. One view is that some of the children with cow's milk allergy do not become milk tolerant, and their allergy persists into adulthood. Another view is that the persistent form of milk allergy may be first realized in early childhood but is immunologically distinct from the much more common childhood milk allergy. The immune reaction in the adult cases that persist is more intense and more specific. This is a hypersensitivity immune condition, meaning even very small amounts of the specific (usually protein) antigen will trigger a significant reaction, and the reactions can be more severe. With a large range of findings, reports say

Report of Michigan Fresh Unprocessed Whole Milk Workgroup

that between 15% and 70% of children with the generic early childhood allergic reaction to milk will maintain the hypersensitivity into adulthood. It is clear that the persistent milk allergy is predominantly hypersensitivity to the casein molecules, but individuals can be triggered by different classes of casein and even the whey proteins (lactoglobulins). Some adults with this form of milk allergy did not exhibit any reaction to milk in their childhood, and some "outgrow" the hypersensitivity later in life.

Nearly all research on milk allergies has used commercial cow's milk. There does not appear to be any study that used fresh unprocessed whole milk. And we are unaware of any collection of reports from persons or newborns drinking fresh unprocessed whole milk that would suggest that the allergic reactions do not occur when the milk is fresh and unprocessed. However, because these immunological reactions are very specific to the configuration of the protein allergen, studies could be conducted to see if milk proteins subject to pasteurization and homogenization, and those native to the unprocessed milk, have the same frequency of allergenic reactions.

Lactose intolerance

Lactose intolerance (also called lactose maldigestion, or lactose malabsorption) adversely affects 10% of the public in the U.S. (15% of households), 29 million Americans. [Opinion Research 2007]

Lactose intolerance is not a disease; it is a condition that arises in some people as they become older. The symptoms are variable amounts of abdominal pain, diarrhea, and intestinal gas. People usually learn that the symptoms occur when they drink milk or consume any dairy product. Lactose is the sugar in milk (of all mammals) and lactose is only present in the milk of mammals. Lactose is most effectively digested by an enzyme lactase (which is a p-galactosidase) forming glucose and galactose. These two sugars are readily absorbed from the small intestine and provide a rapid source of energy (glucose) and a more long-term source of energy (galactose). Lactase is produced by the surface lining cells of the small intestine. As milk is consumed, our intestinal lactase splits the lactose into glucose and galactose which are readily absorbed in the small intestine. In some people, the amount of lactase produced by the lining cells declines as they get older. The amount of reduction is genetically controlled, and varies from person to person, as well as in people with different ethnic backgrounds. If the amount of lactase in the small intestine is not adequate to digest all of the lactose passing through, then the residual continues into the large intestine, which does not produce lactase. Within the large intestine, the complex and variable microflora do digest the residual lactose, but by-products of these processes produce gas, irritate the intestine, and cause the symptoms of the condition.

Due to the fact that some of the lactose in the consumed milk is already digested before it reaches the large intestine by mechanisms other than the intestinal lactase activity, the residual entering the large intestine is reduced. This could happen in the milk prior to consumption, as well as within the transit of the milk after it is consumed. There is a large group of naturally occurring bacteria (many present in the dairy environment) that either digest lactose for their own energy needs, or produce exogenous lactases that digest lactose and produce by-products within the milk. The activity of digesting the lactose by some of these bacteria increases the acidity of the milk. The result of the activity of others is to convert lactose into glucose and galactose, resulting in an increase in the sweetness of the milk. Many exogenous lactases are inactivated by the conditions in the stomach. However, this inactivation is minimized in the presence of milk. If these bacteria are allowed to be present in the milk, and are not inactivated by heating, they will effectively decrease the lactose load.

Susceptible individuals learn to avoid milk and, depending on the severity of their condition, may need to avoid even small amounts of lactose present as ingredients in non-dairy products. The list of foods that contain lactose is very long, and even some prescription medications utilize lactose as an ingredient. There is considerable controversy about the naming of the condition, the diagnostic criteria, and the accuracy of the diagnosis. Consequently, the size of the affected population is also controversial.

There are hundreds of published studies on the prevalence of lactose intolerance. But it is impossible to give a definitive answer to the most obvious question, "How many people have lactose intolerance?" The variability in the reported prevalence is due to differences in population groups, differences in diagnostic criteria, differences in amount of lactose in the challenge dose used, and to some extent the bias of the group performing the study. North American Caucasian populations, for example, have a low percentage; African American have a high percentage. Examples published include: 50%-100% of African Americans, 5%-15% of Caucasian Americans. Almost all current reviews stress that many more people believe that they have lactose intolerant than are diagnosed by laboratory tests. Even with the lowest reported prevalence, there are millions of adults in the U.S. who have this condition. The public health impact from lactose intolerance is not that these people become sick, it is that people who avoid milk because of their lactose intolerance are missing the nutritional benefits of having milk in their diets.

There are testimonials from individuals who had not been drinking milk (because of lactose intolerance), that they are able to regularly drink fresh unprocessed whole milk. To explore this anecdotal information in more detail, an extensive questionnaire was distributed in May 2007 to families that belong to cow share dairy groups in Michigan. Included in the questionnaire were questions about lactose intolerance. Of the 2,500 individuals surveyed, 6% reported having received a professional diagnosis of lactose intolerance. More than 80% of those individuals reported that they did not experience symptoms of lactose intolerance after drinking fresh unprocessed whole milk.

Report of Michigan Fresh Unprocessed Whole Milk Workgroup

While not confirmatory, the results suggest that for, potentially, a large number of people, drinking fresh unprocessed whole milk may represent an alternative to abstaining from milk altogether. The testimonies and findings from this survey do not provide objective criteria of lactose intolerance nor provide an explanation for the findings.

Adulterants

- From feed. Feeds are a potential source of ingredients or contaminants that could end up in the milk produced in cows. Chemicals applied to forage as part of management, in pasture or once harvested, could also contaminate the milk produced in cows.

- Residuals from cleaning operations or pharmaceutical treatment of the cows, as well as drugs used to enhance milk production, can end up in the milk.

Both the public's perception of the consequences of adulterants or residuals, as well as scientific findings of their adverse effects, strongly influence fresh unprocessed whole milk consumer choices.

Report of Michigan Fresh Unprocessed Whole Milk Workgroup

Adverse Consequences Unique to Fresh Unprocessed Whole Milk Consumption

Initial reaction to higher butterfat content
There have been instances in which people have had intestinal reactions when consuming generous servings of fresh whole milk for the first time. There may be a temporary laxative effect. One of the unofficial suggestions is that people trying this milk for the first time should start out drinking small amounts.

Initial reaction to higher concentration of microorganisms
There have been instances in which people have had transitional changes in intestinal reactions to microorganisms when they first start consuming fresh whole milk. One of the interpretations is that this may be a reaction of their intestinal microflora to the input of additional bacteria in the fresh unprocessed whole milk they drank.

Changes in flavors
There are, from time to time, changes in the taste of fresh unprocessed whole milk, related to the feed, condition of the lactating animals, and other factors. Milk readily absorbs smells from the environment, so some flavors may come from milk exposed to the farm, milking area, home, or refrigerator smells. Consumers need to understand that this is to be expected. However, there are times when some or many consumers notice a change in the milk that they find objectionable, that change the way the milk tastes or behaves. Consumers are told that when this happens, they should contact the farmer.

Table of Terms

Word or Phrase	Synonym	Description Particularly Suitable for Discussion of Foodborne Bacterial Pathogens
Biofilm		Some bacteria are able to secrete a biochemical netting that can cover and protect colonies from other bacteria, germicides, and other adverse conditions. When these nettings form on the surface of containers, tubing, or mechanical structures, the biofilm can shield the underlying bacteria. Biofilm is not visible without magnification with a microscope; it is not uncommon for bacteria to grow under biofilm produced by other bacteria.
Carrier state		Person or animal without symptoms of illness that harbors and sheds virulent bacteria that can infect others or contaminate the environment
Challenge dose		In the specific discussion of testing for lactose intolerance, the amount of lactose introduced (ingested) that is used to trigger a response and is then measured by the specific test.
Colonization		Some pathogens are able to grow within the intestinal tract of humans or animals, without causing illness. To distinguish this from infection, when it occurs without illness, it is termed colonization.
Colonizers		When an animal's intestinal tract contains virulent bacteria that are shed in the feces, however, the animal is not ill

Report of Michigan Fresh Unprocessed Whole Milk Workgroup

Word or Phrase	Synonym	Description Particularly Suitable for Discussion of Foodborne Bacterial Pathogens
colony forming units	Cpu	Unit of measure for numbers of bacteria in a sample. Describes the number of colonies that form from a sample. When bacteria multiply on culture, they form masses called colonies. Some bacteria adhere to each other; it is not possible to be sure that each colony results from the multiplication of a single starting bacterium. Therefore, the term colony forming units is used to acknowledge that the origin of the colony could have been a single bacterium or a group of bacteria that were stuck together.
Compete		Ability of a specific type of bacteria to grow/multiply when surrounded by other types in the same environment
Competitive Inhibition	Competitive Exclusion	Within many environments there are large numbers of different bacteria, many of which are present in very large numbers. In such complex environments, those bacteria present in small numbers grow more slowly or may be excluded. There are many explanations for this inhibition, including the ability of some bacteria to secrete products that kill or injure other bacteria, the competition for nutrients, and physical interactions.
Culture		Laboratory technique to enable individual bacteria present in a specimen to grow/multiply forming masses/colonies visible to the unaided eye. Also a mixture of nutrients specifically formulated to enable specific types of bacteria to grow/multiply.

Report of Michigan Fresh Unprocessed Whole Milk Workgroup

Word or Phrase	Synonym	Description Particularly Suitable for Discussion of Foodborne Bacterial Pathogens
Endemic		A specific disease occurrence that is widespread across a large geographic area. Usually pertaining to a single animal or group of animals.
Enteritis	Gastro-enteritis	Illness involving the cells lining the intestinal tract, including the stomach, small, and large intestine.
Epidemic		Disease that is a significant public health problem spreading and infecting large numbers of people, or specific animals.
Epidemic clones		Occasionally, an outbreak occurs with unusually high numbers of severe illness complications. The strain identified is often called an epidemic clone. Most commonly used with listeriosis.
Exogenous	extracellular	Exogenous toxins are those that are active outside of the bacteria that produce the toxin. Endogenous toxins remain inside the body of the bacterium. In the context of lactose intolerance, exogenous enzymes are active outside of the intestinal cells or bacteria that produced them. Endogenous enzymes function within the body of the bacterium.
Extrapulmonary		Localized disease in parts of the body other than the airways and lungs

Report of Michigan Fresh Unprocessed Whole Milk Workgroup

Word or Phrase	Synonym	Description Particularly Suitable for Discussion of Foodborne Bacterial Pathogens
Filter	Inline Filter (sock filter) Milk Filter	Membrane filter in the pipe lines from the milking to the bulk storage tank, designed to remove particles from the milk
Flagella		A specific type of thread-like projection from the cell wall of some types of bacteria that enable movement
Flagellar serotypes	"H" antigens	Category of subtypes distinguished by the proteins in the bacteria's flagellum. Testing is made easier since the characteristic is on the outside of the bacteria.
Forage		Natural animal feed composed of grasses and non-woody plants as eaten in pasture, or harvested as hay. Generally does not include the seeds or roots.
Fresh, Unprocessed Whole Milk	FUW Milk	The product intended for direct human consumption since "raw milk" is used to describe milk intended for pasteurization.
Gastroenteritis	Enteritis, gastro-intestinal Illness	Illness involving the cells lining the intestinal tract, including the stomach, small, and large intestine.
Genus		Scientifically established subgroup under "Family". The genus name is the first word in the official name for a bacterial group, e.g., *Listeria monocytogenes*. Listeria is the genus, monocytogenes is the species.

Report of Michigan Fresh Unprocessed Whole Milk Workgroup

Word or Phrase	Synonym	Description Particularly Suitable for Discussion of Foodborne Bacterial Pathogens
Gram negative		Large group of bacteria identified under the microscope because they stain "negative" with dyes included in the Gram Stain. After the method is complete, individual bacteria have a pink color.
Gram positive		Large group of bacteria identified under the microscope because they stain "positive" with dyes included in the Gram Stain. After the method is complete, individual bacteria have a purple color.
H (serotypes)	Flagellar antigens	A protein associated with flagella (projections on surface of bacteria that enable motility), easily identified by commercially available tests and used to distinguish between serotypes of bacteria, e.g., *E. coli* H7.
Hemolytic uremic syndrome	HUS	Serious complication associated with certain forms of toxins produced by some virulent bacteria that may cause temporary kidney failure, particularly in children.
Horizontal transfer	Lateral Transgenic	Genetic information that has been transferred between different species, usually with viruses acting as the transfer agent. In contrast to ancestral genetic information. Genetic material that has been passed down over a long period of time from generation to generation. The DNA is within a chromosome. See sidebar in Pathogen Summary -*E. coli* page 70.

Report of Michigan Fresh Unprocessed Whole Milk Workgroup

Word or Phrase	Synonym	Description Particularly Suitable for Discussion of Foodborne Bacterial Pathogens
Host adapted		A particular subtype of bacteria that has become selectively virulent in a single animal. Does not grow or multiply in other animals.
Immunity	resistance	General term used to describe mechanisms that resist infection
Incubation times		Interval between ingestion of virulent bacteria and onset of symptoms of illness
Infectious dose		Amount of a virulent bacteria that will cause illness when consumed. See Discussion of Infectious Dose.
Infectious	virulent	Capable of establishing physical location to grow and multiply in a host. Also meaning a form of bacteria that can be spread from one infected individual to others.
Inoculated		Mechanically introduce a type of bacteria. Usually in the context of an experiment to determine fate of a specific type of bacteria. Example: inoculating 100,000 individual bacteria into milk to determine whether they will grow, multiply, become inactivated, or are killed.
Intercellular space	interstitial	In tissues, the space between cells.
Intestinal microflora		The complex of microorganism that populate the gut. Includes all forms of microscopic organisms.

Word or Phrase	Synonym	Description Particularly Suitable for Discussion of Foodborne Bacterial Pathogens
Intracellular obligate parasite		Organism that will only grow within living cells of the host animal
Isolate		Specific bacteria that originate from a single cultured colony, considered to all be identical to the bacteria that multiplied to form the colony
Lineage		Grouping of bacterial subtypes generally related to genetic heritage
Listerosis		In general, any illness caused by listeria. However, it is more commonly used to describe the extremely rare, severe systemic illness, excluding the far more frequent mild forms of gastroenteritis.
Mastitis		Any infection of the mammary glands
Milk Ring Test	brucella milk ring test (BRT)	Screening test for brucella infection in dairy herds producing milk
Matching		Some significant laboratory evidence that two or more isolates/strains of bacteria were the "same" or very similar
Motile		Capable of self-propelled movement, usually determined by observing the bacteria with a microscope

Word or Phrase	Synonym	Description Particularly Suitable for Discussion of Foodborne Bacterial Pathogens
O (serotypes)	somatic antigens	Technically, a portion of a large molecule embedded in the cell wall of bacteria. Differences in this portion of the molecule are used to distinguish subtypes of bacteria. Commercial reagents enable rapid identification of the different subtypes, e.g., *E. coli* O157 is number 157 in the list of different 0 antigens which have been identified in different subtypes of *E. coli*.
Obligate parasite		Will only grow and multiply within the cells of a host
Outbreak		Technically, two or more illnesses in people that are linked by a common source and within a specified time course
Pathogen		General term for group of bacteria that have been associated with illness. Usually in the form of the scientific name for the group.
Perinatal illness		Illness that occurs during the development of the fetus and in the newborn
Persistent carrier state		Continuing to shed virulent bacteria for a long time (years) after an infection, but without symptoms of illness.
Rod shaped	Rod-shaped	Bacteria with elongated body when viewed in the microscope. In contrast to cocci which are spherically shaped.

Report of Michigan Fresh Unprocessed Whole Milk Workgroup

Word or Phrase	Synonym	Description Particularly Suitable for Discussion of Foodborne Bacterial Pathogens
Ruminant animals		Sub-classification of animals (including cows, goats, and sheep) that have a digestive system that efficiently digests grasses and hay (leafy plants high in cellulose fiber)
Secondary Infection	Secondary Illness	Within a cluster of illnesses associated with a common cause; when someone becomes infected from close contact with someone in the cluster, rather than from ingesting the food, they are categorized as secondary infections. In contrast, those who become infected from consumption of the food are considered primary infections.
Self-limiting		Illness resolves without medical interventions.
Serotype	serovar	Category of subtypes distinguishable by different protein antigens (typically distinguished by the use of commercial antibody preparations)
Serovar	Serotype	Subtype distinguishable by different antigens (typically distinguished by the use of commercial antibody preparations). This is used with subtypes of the genus salmonella. In most other organisms, the term serotype is used to distinguish subtypes of a species based on differences in a surface protein on the organism.

Word or Phrase	Synonym	Description Particularly Suitable for Discussion of Foodborne Bacterial Pathogens
Somatic antigen		Characteristic of an antigen contained within the body, of a bacterium
Species		Scientifically established subgroup under "Genus". The species name is the second word in the official name for a bacterial group, e.g., *Listeria monocytogenes*. Listeria is the genus, monocytogenes is the species
Sporadic cases	isolated cases	In epidemiology, this describes those individuals with illness that have no known association with other ill individuals.
spp		When used in a scientific name the scientific abbreviation tor "all species" e.g. *Salmonella spp.* Meaning all of the species within the genus salmonella.
Strains	subtypes	A term used for subtypes of a species
Subclinical		Infectious state when the outward signs of illness are minimal
Subspecies		Recognized subdivisions of the named species
Subtype	Substrain	General term used to describe different groups within a named species

Report of Michigan Fresh Unprocessed Whole Milk Workgroup

Word or Phrase	Synonym	Description Particularly Suitable for Discussion of Foodborne Bacterial Pathogens
Super-Shedders		When there is colonization of pathogens in the intestines of animals, the condition is generally transient and the concentration of pathogens shed in the feces is low. However, there are uncommon individual animals that tend to have persistent colonization and shed much higher concentrations of the pathogen in their feces. These individual animals are called super-shedders.
Susceptible		Person who is capable of becoming infected
Systemic disease	widespread	The infectious bacteria have spread from the intestine into the body, usually through the blood stream, and may infect other organs of the body.
tolerant	transient	In the context of allergic milk reactions, tolerant describes the finding that some people with milk allergies find that, at a later time, they no longer react to milk. Some people contrast persistent cow's milk allergy with transient/tolerant forms.
Toxin		Molecule, often a protein, produced by bacteria that cause damage or illness. Some bacterial toxins remain within the bacteria (endogenous), while others are secreted outside (exogenous).

Report of Michigan Fresh Unprocessed Whole Milk Workgroup

Word or Phrase	Synonym	Description Particularly Suitable for Discussion of Foodborne Bacterial Pathogens
Transient colonization	Temporary intestinal colonizers	Some pathogens are able to grow within the intestinal tract of humans or animals, without causing illness. When this colonization occurs for only a short time, or intermittently, it is termed transient. The usual pattern in these cases is that the concentration of pathogens shed in the feces is low.
Unprocessed milk	raw milk	Milk that has not been pasteurized, homogenized, separated, or otherwise mechanically altered after milking
Virulence factors		Individual component of a virulent bacteria necessary in the sequence of steps leading to illness
Virulent		Technical term describing the ability of a specific subtype of bacteria that have the genetic information necessary to cause illness
zoonotic		Infectious diseases transmitted to humans from infected animals. Occasionally applied to human infections transmitted from animals, even if the animals were not sick.

Topic 4

Risk and Benefit Management

1. What steps are necessary to minimize the health risk for consumers of fresh unprocessed whole milk?

2. Who is responsible for minimizing risk, as it relates to fresh unprocessed whole milk?

3. What steps can be taken to mitigate or prevent adverse impacts on the entire dairy industry in the event of a milkborne outbreak originating from milk consumption?

4. What management practices enhance benefits?

Summary

Approved August 28, 2012

Topic 4 – Risk and Benefit Management

Introduction

In addressing the Working Group's Topic: Risk & Benefit Management questions 1 and 2—**"What steps are necessary to minimize the health risk for consumers of fresh unprocessed whole milk?" and "Who is responsible for minimizing risk, as it relates to fresh unprocessed whole milk?"**—we built on information and discussions in the previous topics, with additional information from consumers and practicing farmers. The group is not suggesting that the guidelines should be associated with a certification process, regulatory standards, and/or "best practices". The working group decided that we would provide guidelines, not propose rules/regulations, goals, or requirements. And as we progressed through an orderly review of the risks, we determined that the guidelines would be best expressed in general terms. We also decided that providing these guidelines by listing columns for "Issues/Concerns", "Management Practices", "(How)", "Why", and "Who", in the form of a table, would facilitate understanding of our summaries. The text in each box is intended to suggest areas of management and are intentionally brief, rather than detailed and specific. The items in the table, Risk Management Summary, are grouped in categories; however, there is no intent to list by priority or importance. These are a set of guidelines that should assist the farmer and consumer when considering their practices and management choices. We are unable to document evidence that would enable ranking the importance of the guidelines, nor to determine that any guideline is the optimal way to avoid risk.

The guidelines go beyond the traditional items included in risk management of food production. Typically, such lists focus almost entirely on mitigating consumer illnesses. The market for Fresh Unprocessed Whole Milk (FUW milk) is driven largely by consumer demand for this product. Some of the items are based on recognition of some of the specific factors important to current consumers in Michigan—including factors that they want, and those that they do not want. Our group did not attempt to determine the rationale for these consumer preferences, other than accepting that they strongly influence current consumer choice for this product. And because the production of FUW milk is primarily consumer driven, and certain dairy practices are unacceptable to these consumers, we expanded our listing to include items that could result in loss of consumers. We also expanded our listing to include items concerning the health of the dairy animals.

Our summary makes the important point that risk management is the responsibility of all those that handle FUW milk, including farmers, handlers, and consumers.

Report of Michigan Fresh Unprocessed Whole Milk Workgroup

Our group recognizes that it is not possible to actually determine that any of the items in the table have a proven record of reducing associated health risk. As shown in the Workgroup's Topic: Risks, since the total numbers of clusters of illnesses attributed to the consumption of FUW milk (the Workgroup agreed to use the term fresh unprocessed whole milk, or FUW milk, to describe the product intended for direct human consumption since "raw milk" is used to describe milk intended for pasteurization) is small, investigations of these incidents have not determined a specific practice that might have been responsible for transmitting the infections. In many cases, dairies that were associated with a cluster of illnesses have continued to supply FUW milk without any recurrence of illnesses in their consumers. There is some research on linking specific practices to the transmission of infections, but none specifically using FUW milk. Nearly all traditional mitigation suggestions are based on actions that might, theoretically, influence foodborne infections. However, we are unable to find any documentation of actual reduction in the rate of clusters of illnesses attributed to FUW milk when specific practices were changed. Therefore, it is important for farmers and consumers to understand that following the guidelines in the table below, either entirely or individually, will not guarantee that the produced and consumed milk will never be a vehicle for milkborne illnesses. The Workgroup does not imply that production, handling, and consumption of milk following these guidelines will result in fewer illnesses and certainly they are not an assurance/guarantee that the milk will always be safe. Nothing can guarantee that any food is always safe.

These guidelines considered conditions as they exist in Michigan in 2012. These will most likely evolve as producers, consumers, and researchers learn more about Fresh Unprocessed Whole Milk.

Table of Risk Management

HYGIENE

Issue/Concern	Management Practice	Why	Who
Keep dairy housing clean	Have a management plan to keep housing areas clean	Consumer choice and animal health	Farmer
Wear clean outer garments	Use footwear and coveralls appropriate to areas of operations	Minimize contamination with high concentrations of pathogens virulent in people. Consumer preference	All
Keep milking and milk handling areas clean	Regular cleaning and good housekeeping	Consumer choice, animal health and minimizing contamination	Farmer, Consumer
Keep equipment and containers clean	Regular cleaning	Consumer choice, animal health and minimizing contamination	Farmer, Consumer
Separate source of water from dairy animals	Avoid animals contaminating water supplies	Consumer choice and animal health	Farmer

Report of Michigan Fresh Unprocessed Whole Milk Workgroup

CONSUMER PREFERENCES

Issue/Concern	Management Practice	Why	Who
Providing undesirable feed	Choice of feed	Change taste of milk or how milk can be used	Farmer
Undesirable ingredients in feed	Choice of feed	Consumer wants to avoid certain ingredients in feed	Farmer
Lack of communication between farmer and consumer/ written agreement	Have a formal contract between farmer and consumer	Many reasons	Farmer, Consumer
Consumer rejection of products	Respond to consumer's desires about feed and animal treatments	Consumer choice	Farmer
Do not import milk from another dairy	Only use milk from your dairy animals	Consumer choice. Trace back is severely compromised. Increased risks from management of other dairy	Farmer
Labeling as milk	Labeling	Ensure that consumers know that it is fresh unprocessed whole milk	Farmer
Maintain creamline	Do not separate out cream from milk, give appropriate feed, and select herd genetics	Consumers will want to have cream and assurance the milk is not degraded	Farmer
Real-time communication between farmer and consumer	Provisions in contract form; establish trust and personal interactions	Feedback on changes in milk: taste/smell, ability to make products, adverse reactions, and speed of trace back and recall when necessary	Farmer, Consumer

Report of Michigan Fresh Unprocessed Whole Milk Workgroup

DAIRY ANIMALS

Issue/Concern	Management Practice	Why	Who
Check quality of feed supplier	Know feed supplier and monitor quality of any feed	Feed can be a source of infectious agents or toxic contaminants	Farmer
Maximize forage and grain	Utilize pasture	Animal health and quality of milk are optimized if appropriate feed is supplied. Consumers have preferences	Farmer
High quality feed	Pasture. Optimize forage types and quality to suit animal/genetics	Optimize animal health, quality of milk produced. Consumers are often very concerned about animal nutrition	Farmer
Use local feed sources	Purchase feed locally	Influence consumer choice	Farmer
Keeping beneficial biology of intestinal tract	Manage quality of feed	Feed choice influences intestinal tract biology	Farmer
Keeping soil in balance	Ongoing soil monitoring including microbiology	Feed choice influences intestinal tract biology	Farmer
Keeping soil organic content high	Monitor soils and augment with appropriate organic material	Improve quality of feed	Farmer
Maintain quality of imported feed	Ensure that imported feeds are of high quality	Animal health	Farmer

Report of Michigan Fresh Unprocessed Whole Milk Workgroup

DAIRY ANIMALS

Issue/Concern	Management Practice	Why	Who
Improving soils	Test soils, soil plan	Improve quality of feed	Farmer
Avoid animal stress	Attention to farm design and management	Consumers are concerned about animal welfare. Stress can adversely affect animal health	Farmer
Cleaning up manure	Avoid accumulation of manure	Animal health and consumer concern about farm management and milk quality	Farmer
Closed herd	Maintain closed herd	Consumer choice and animal health	Farmer
Control herd genetics, for example, butterfat, protein, and animal health	Develop herd genetics	Animal health, animal stress, and milk quality	Farmer
Colostrum	Segregate milk from dairy animals that recently calved	Colostrum is not milk	Farmer, Consumer
Keep herd small in number	Management choice	Keep operations manageable, minimize infectious diseases in herd	Farmer

Report of Michigan Fresh Unprocessed Whole Milk Workgroup

DAIRY ANIMALS

Issue/Concern	Management Practice	Why	Who
Lactation management	Avoid late lactation milk	Farmer preference. Potential adverse taste of milk	Farmer
Milkings per day	Decide on frequency of milkings	Farmer preference	Farmer
Maintain adequate ventilation	Design barn with good ventilation	Animal health and consumer concern about farm management	Farmer
Minimize confinement of dairy animals	Make choices on design of stalls	Consumers are concerned about animal welfare. Design of stall influences dairy animals' behavior, cleanliness, stress	Farmer
Provide clean bedding	Maintain clean area for animals to bed, both indoors and outdoors	Animal health and consumer concern about farm management	Farmer
Keep milk from suspect dairy animals separate	Identify unhealthy dairy animals and keep their milk separate	Human health	Farmer
Reduce contact with fresh manure	Keep environment, housing, animals, containers, equipment, and people handling milk, clean	Consumer choice and animal health. Keep milk visibly clean for consumer acceptance	Farmer

Report of Michigan Fresh Unprocessed Whole Milk Workgroup

MILK

Issue/Concern	Management Practice	Why	Who
Filter milk	Filter milk	Avoid clumps of material that might contain high concentrations of undesirable bacteria	Farmer
Chill milk immediately	Chill milk immediately to 42°F or less within 45 minutes of milking	Maintain levels and types of microorganisms in milk, maintain taste and shelf life	Farmer
Evenly distribute butterfat	Keep cream evenly suspended when filling consumers' containers	Consumers want the cream	Farmer, Handler, Consumer
Keep milk cold	After chilling, maintain at 35°F to 38°F through distribution and home storage until milk is consumed	Extend shelf life. Maintain microbiological balance in milk. Minimize enzymatic and other undesirable concentrations in the milk	Farmer, Handler, Consumer
Do not keep milk at refrigerated temperatures for months	Suggest 'consume by' time	Avoid growth of listeria and other undesirable microorganisms that might increase to undesirable concentrations in the milk.	Farmer, Consumer

Report of Michigan Fresh Unprocessed Whole Milk Workgroup

MILK

Issue/Concern	Management Practice	Why	Who
Maintain open and trusting relationship between farmer and consumer	Formalize agreement (contract) while keeping a personal relationship. Maintain reliable and rapid means of communication between consumers and farmers	The consumer is a valuable monitor of the quality of the milk. Since they consume and use their milk regularly, changes in the taste/smell, appearance, and the way it behaves (including shelf life and ability to make products) are more likely to be noticed. If there is an open and trusting relationship it is more likely that undesirable changes in the milk will be recognized and addressed.	Farmer, Consumer
Distribute to a well-defined consumer pool	Formalize agreement (contract). Encourage trust. Maintain personal contact	The ability to trace problems, identify causes of any problems and facilitate rapid and effective corrective action is enhanced	Farmer, Consumer
Initial reaction to drinking FUW milk	When drinking FUW milk for the first time, consume in moderation	Consumption of any new food product can lead to gastrointestinal issues	Consumer

Report of Michigan Fresh Unprocessed Whole Milk Workgroup

MONITORING, LABORATORY TESTING, AND RECORD-KEEPING

Issue/Concern	Management Practice	Why	Who
Cull persistent high shedders	Monitor for pathogens in animals; if individual dairy animals are positive, they should be removed from the farm	Dairy animals may be colonized with pathogens, but usually only for a short period, shedding low concentrations of those pathogens. However, colonization rarely persists and these individuals may shed higher concentrations. They are potential sources of contamination of the herd, and the farm environment	Farmer
Maintain records, observations, animal health	Monitor, save	Enable quality control management. Promote transparency. Enhance consumer confidence	Farmer
Monitoring animal behavior	Observe animals for behavior suggestive of listeriosis	To avoid listeriosis in herd	Farmer

Report of Michigan Fresh Unprocessed Whole Milk Workgroup

MONITORING, LABORATORY TESTING, AND RECORD-KEEPING

Issue/Concern	Management Practice	Why	Who
Monitoring animal behavior and vaccinations	Test for bovine viruses or vaccinate	Maintain herd health	Farmer
Observe animals in herd	Observation of behavior; testing with somatic cell count (SCC)	Herd and individual animal health, to enable prompt and appropriate interventions	Farmer
Testing animals upon entering herd	Test all new animals entering the herd for bovine tuberculosis, brucella, Johnes	To avoid communicable diseases in herd	Farmer
Decreasing environmental contaminants	Monitor farm environment, avoid contamination of farm with biological, chemical, and physical hazards	Animal health	Farmer
Testing/record maintenance	Test, monitor, save, and display records	Enable quality control management. Promote transparency. Enhance consumer confidence	Farmer
Adverse event	Develop and maintain a written plan to address an adverse event that may occur	A rapid response and evaluation may minimize potential consequence of adverse event.	Farmer

Report of Michigan Fresh Unprocessed Whole Milk Workgroup

SOURCES OF PATHOGENS VIRULENT IN PEOPLE

Issue/Concern	Management Practice	Why	Who
Vigorous cleaning of equipment	Monitor for bacteria in milk by using one of the available tests. Watch for high spikes of bacterial counts. If cause of these spikes cannot be easily explained and corrective action taken, then vigorously clean the milking, milk handling, and milk storage equipment	Many microorganisms in milk are able to form biofilm, which are sequestered and persistent environments for proliferation of microorganisms. When biofilm with masses of bacteria become free in the milk, they can be a source of periodic high spikes in bacteria counts in the milk. Biofilm is difficult to remove, without aggressive cleaning, including mechanical brushing	Farmer
Keep high concentrations of virulent pathogens from containers	Avoid contamination of milk containers with high concenrations of pathogens virulent in people. This includes keeping sick people from handling containers.	Milk containers can transmit infectious bacteria if the contamination is with high concentrations and the time after contamination is short.	Farmer, Handler, Consumer

---

Report of Michigan Fresh Unprocessed Whole Milk Workgroup

126

SOURCES OF PATHOGENS VIRULENT IN PEOPLE

Issue/Concern	Management Practice	Why	Who
Keep people with virulent pathogens from contact with milk	Sick people, particulary those with diarrheal infections, must avoid contact with farm animals, milking operations, handling of milk and milk containers.	Because these people shed high concentrations of virulent microorganisms that are virulent in people. Avoid contamination with high concentrations of microorganisms that are virulent in people.	Farmer, Handler, Consumer
Avoid contamination of milk with infectious material from poultry processing	Separate milk handling operations from poultry processing/butchering operations.	Poultry intestinal tracts commonly contain high concentrations of pathogens that could infect people. During processing the pathogens could contaminate milk being handled in the same area.	Farmer
Separate calves from dairy animals	Birthing area and young dairy animals should be kept in an area away from the dairy herd.	Although colonization with pathogens is transient and shedding is with low numbers, it has been shown that calves may have a higher prevalence of colonization, and shed with higher numbers of pathogens.	Farmer

Report of Michigan Fresh Unprocessed Whole Milk Workgroup

SOURCES OF PATHOGENS VIRULENT IN PEOPLE

Issue/Concern	Management Practice	Why	Who
Separate dairy animals from poultry	Minimize co-mingling of poultry with dairy animals. If poultry are present, the flock should be tested for shedding of pathogens virulent in people.	Poultry are a common source of high concentrations of pathogens. If the pathogens are virulent in people, the poultry can be source of colonization in dairy animals.	Farmer
Separate milking and storage of milk areas from poultry	Minimize co-mingling of poultry with dairy animals, milking operations, and milk handling areas. If poultry are present, the flock should be tested for shedding of pathogens virulent in people.	Poultry are a common source of high concentrations of pathogens. If the pathogens are virulent in people, the poultry can be source of colonization in dairy animals, direct contamination of milk and containers with numbers of virulent pathogens that could infect consumers.	Farmer
Separate farm animals	Design and eqip facilities to separate groups of farm animals.	To minimize the spread of potential virulent pathogens.	Farmer

SOURCES OF PATHOGENS VIRULENT IN PEOPLE

Issue/Concern	Management Practice	Why	Who
Separation of poultry from areas where milk containers are filled	Minimize co-mingling of poultry with dairy animals, milking operations, and milk handling areas. If poultry are present, the flock should be tested for shedding of pathogens virulent in people. Poultry should be kept out of areas where milk containers are filled.	Poultry are a common source of high concentrations of pathogens. If the pathogens are virulent in people, the poultry can be source of colonization in dairy animals, direct contamination of milk and containers with numbers of virulent pathogens that could infect consumers.	Farmer, Handler, Consumer
Avoid handling milk in areas of the home where fresh meat and poultry has been handled	If fresh meat and poultry has been handled in the kitchen, the surfaces and utilities should be cleaned before milk is handled in the same area, or by the same people.	Fresh meats are a common risk of pathogens in high concentrations. Fluids in the packaging can contaminate surfaces, equipment and people.	Consumer
Cull individual animals	Monitor herd	Animal health, improve handling of animals	Farmer

Report of Michigan Fresh Unprocessed Whole Milk Workgroup

WATER

Issue/Concern	Management Practice	Why	Who
Cleaning before milking	Clean teats before milking. Avoid accumulation of dirt on dairy animals	Animal health	Farmer
Ensuring that irrigation water is clean	If irrigation is necessary, avoid using contaminated water	Animal health	Farmer
Keeping dairy animals out of water	Separate dairy animals from standing water	Animal health	Farmer
Keeping manure out of water	Separate dairy animals from standing water	Animal health	Farmer
Locating the well away from sources of contamination	Avoid contamination of well water	Well water is used in cleaning	Farmer
Maintain clean, fresh water supply for animals	Monitor with testing of all water supplies	Water is essential for animal health. Water can be contaminated without visible change	Farmer
Testing water for contamination	Monitor with testing of all water supplies	Water is essential for animal health. Water can be contaminated without visible change	Farmer

Report of Michigan Fresh Unprocessed Whole Milk Workgroup

Question 3. What steps can be taken to mitigate or prevent adverse impacts on the entire dairy industry in the event of a milkborne outbreak originating from milk consumption?

The Workgroup encourages more people to include milk in their regular diet and is concerned about factors that would reduce the public's perception of the benefits of milk. Both the advocates for fresh unprocessed whole milk and organized dairy are eager to increase the consumption of milk.

The risk that there will be a reduction of consumption of conventional milk if we enable raw milk (FUW milk) production –
An independent survey conducted in Michigan found that many people who are currently obtaining fresh unprocessed whole milk (FUW milk) want to include milk in their diet, but do not want the product that is widely available in the retail markets. Many of those using herd share operations to obtain FUW milk were not previously drinking conventional milk. Enabling these people to consume a product (FUW milk) enhances the mutual goal of having more people include milk in their diet. The Workgroup is not aware of any evidence that making FUW milk available reduces the market for conventional milk.

The risk that there will be a reduction in the conventional milk market resulting from announcements of foodborne outbreaks attributed to raw milk (FUW milk) –
There is accumulating evidence that there is a reduction in the market for a category of food that is the target of an ongoing investigation of illnesses. This has been documented for incidents in which media attention accompanying public health announcements is widespread and continues over a period of time.

Several factors are associated with this adverse impact on the public's purchasing patterns.
1. Initial public health investigations have progressed to the point that a category of food is strongly suspected as the vehicle for the spread of illnesses, and this prompts mentioning a particular food category in the public notice and media reports.
2. The illnesses occur over a large or unspecified portion of the country, prompting widespread (both regional and national) and sustained media attention.
3. Illnesses continue to be reported well after the index cases, prompting repeated announcements about the suspect food category and continuing media attention which causes general alarm to the public.
4. There is a "recall" of the suspect food category, visible in the retail stores.
5. During the height of the media attention, the investigation has not narrowed the source of the illnesses to a specific product or producer.
6. Despite specificity in the updated agency news releases, the media attention sometimes fails to make it clear that only a subset of the food

Report of Michigan Fresh Unprocessed Whole Milk Workgroup

category is suspected and other supplies of the food are not implicated. The public alarm grows and the public attributes the threat to a food, not a product or producer.

Even though marketing research has shown that the adverse impact on sales is only temporary, even a temporary impact could have significant market risk for the dairy industry since milk has nationwide sales and is frequently and consistently purchased by many households—milk is one of the most common items in the consumer's grocery cart.

However, there are several factors that differentiate the marketing impact of milkborne illnesses from the recent incidents with fruit, leafy crops, nuts, and meat:

- Incidents attributed to raw milk are local because the producer's distribution is geographically very limited, particularly with herd share operations.
- Analysis of incidents attributed to raw milk show that most have a very short media time span—typically several days or a week.
- We are not aware of a milkborne outbreak that was not quickly associated with the specific product and a specific producer. Therefore, the initial, and often only, announcements target raw milk specifically and identify a specific producer.
- Over the last decades the public has learned that "raw milk" is a different product than the commercial milk that they see and purchase in the grocery stores. Public announcements and the resulting media attention have consistently and specifically emphasized the product distinction in all coverage. When raw milk is suspected, no one fails to make the public aware that this is raw milk and not the product Grade "A" pasteurized milk that they are purchasing.

With milk, the possible marketing risk is not theoretical. We have actual experience which enables objective observations. There have not been any scientifically controlled studies on the market effect of raw milk outbreak coverage. But it is difficult to imagine that the public's awareness of raw milk outbreaks can increase above the current dramatic attention that occurs with every incident that is attributed to raw milk. And many of the news releases from government agencies are designed to heighten the public's worry about becoming ill from dairy products that have not been pasteurized.

Report of Michigan Fresh Unprocessed Whole Milk Workgroup

4. What management practices enhance benefits?

Fresh Unprocessed Whole Milk has inherent benefits to the consumer and the farmer. There are certain practices that are understood to preserve and enhance these benefits. Many of these benefits are described in **Topic 2 – Benefits and Values: Question 6. Assuming that all milk is not the same, what do production and management practices have to do with fresh unprocessed whole milk's nutritional value, pathogens, color, taste, etc.?** and Question 7. **What is the impact of consumer preferences on production and management practices of fresh unprocessed whole milk?**

Table of Benefit Management

BENEFITS	PRACTICES

Beneficial Bacteria in FUW Milk	Pasture-based living conditions
	   – Exposure to a variety of fresh, high quality forages contribute to a balanced and diverse population of bacteria and enables reduced grain feeding
	Maintain appropriate level of the ration as forage
	   – High forage intake helps keep the rumen healthy
	A healthy animal
	   – Balanced soils, quality feed, and well managed living conditions promote normal bacteria
	Keep milk cold
	   – Maintains existing balance of bacteria

Enzymes	A healthy animal cold – Balanced soils, quality feed, and excellent living conditions promote a healthy animal
CLAs, Omega 3s (Beneficial Fatty Acids)	Minimal grain feeding – Ample fresh forage and minimal grain promote well balanced fatty acid chains

Report of Michigan Fresh Unprocessed Whole Milk Workgroup

Table of Benefit Management

BENEFITS	PRACTICES
Flavor	Introduce new feeds slowly cold - This keeps the rumen balance and the milk consistent Limit noxious aromatic feeds, especially the turnip and onion families - The butterfat in milk transfers flavor from the diet General cleanliness - Milk takes flavors from its surroundings - Unclean equipment will overwhelm desirable flavors Keep milk cold - Cold milk retains good flavor
Understanding and Appreciation of Milk	Education - Be willing to spend time with consumers to answer questions and make suggestions - Self-education makes for a better relationship and a more rewarding experience Encourage home processing - Home processing fosters appreciation of all processing and a better understanding of the medium Give access to the farm - Regular exposure to the farm and its workings will encourage a greater understanding of milk

Report of Michigan Fresh Unprocessed Whole Milk Workgroup

Table of Benefit Management

BENEFITS	PRACTICES

Consumer Confidence	Give access to the farm
	  - If the consumer is pleased with the farm, it increases confidence in dairy
	Build relationships
	  - Familiarity makes input and concerns more comfortable
	Test cold
	  - Milk consistently documented as clean gives confidence to the consumer as well as the producer
	General cleanliness

Traceability	Testing of milk cold
	  - A consistent testing program can help identify potential problems if there are changes from established patterns
	Organize a regular pickup day with contact information
	  - Consumers can easily be alerted of impure milk
	  - Troubleshooting is simplified
	  - Accurate record-keeping facilitates identification of shareholders

Vitamins and Minerals	Sun exposure increases Vitamin D content

Report of Michigan Fresh Unprocessed Whole Milk Workgroup

Topic 5

Consumer Choice Options

1. How might consumer access to fresh unprocessed whole milk be achieved?

2. How might people who are considering choosing to drink fresh unprocessed whole milk be properly educated and informed on their choice?

Summary

Approved August 28, 2012

Topic 5 – Consumer Choice Options

1. How might consumer access to fresh unprocessed whole milk be achieved?

Based on the attitudes of current consumers of fresh unprocessed whole (FUW) milk, the following was surmised.

Currently, consumers of FUW milk go to great lengths to get their milk. Many make weekly trips out to the farm, taking their own bottles and filling them from the cooled milk supply. Some carpool to share this responsibility, however many are making the weekly trip alone. Others make weekly trips to dedicated drop-off points, including farmers markets, where they can pick up their weekly allotment of their cow share.

Although the consumers of FUW milk understand the restrictions to access of this product and are willing to do what it takes to obtain it, many expressed a desire to be able to purchase milk in a retail setting.

They are frustrated by what they see as unnecessary restrictions to this product and outright prohibition of their ability to make their own food choices.

At this point in time, consumers believe that until the government is willing to objectively look at the data which clearly shows that the risk of drinking FUW milk is relatively nil, consumers are content to continue with the present arrangements of the herd share program. They are also anxious to know that this arrangement will be acceptable to the state so that they and the farmers can be confident about their access to FUW milk. Many expressed the need for more farmers to participate in this program, increasing the supply as well as giving farmers the opportunity to have a successful business by meeting the demand.

2. How might people who are considering choosing to drink fresh unprocessed whole milk be properly educated and informed on their choice?

Government policy should not prevent consumers from making responsible food choices. Educating the consumer about FUW milk should really be the consumer's responsibility. Just as it is the consumer's freedom to decide if they want to smoke cigarettes, drink alcohol, take medications, eat sushi, consume artificial sweeteners, drink espresso, eat soy products, eat GMO foods, or eat a vegan diet/hi carb diet/ animal protein diet. Consumers make these decisions every day. Choices about food

Report of Michigan Fresh Unprocessed Whole Milk Workgroup

are essential to our health and well-being. There is plenty of information available to the consumer who is looking for it on the benefits and risks of drinking FUW milk.

Report of Michigan Fresh Unprocessed Whole Milk Workgroup

Food Safety & Inspection Program

SECTION: General Policy # 1.40 Date: 3/12/2013
Fresh Unprocessed Whole Milk Date: 31/12/2013

Policy

This policy is built upon the recommendations of the Fresh Unprocessed Whole Milk Workgroup. The Workgroup agreed to use the term Fresh Unprocessed Whole (FUW) milk to describe the product intended for direct human consumption since "raw milk" is used to describe milk intended for pasteurization.

Michigan Dairy Laws state in MCL 288.538 and in MCL 288.696, "Only pasteurized milk and milk products shall be offered for sale or sold, directly or indirectly, to the final consumer or to restaurants, grocery stores, or similar establishments." The Food Law states in MCL 289.6140, "Only pasteurized ingredients from a department-approved source shall be used for milk and milk products manufactured, sold, served, or prepared at a retail food establishment."

In a herd share operation, consumers pay a farmer a fee for boarding their animal (or a share of an animal), caring for the animal and milking the animal. The herd share shareholder then obtains (but does not purchase) the raw milk from his or her own animal.

Herd share operations include the following elements.

- There should be a signed and dated written contract between a single herd share farmer and shareholder
- There must be a workable means of communication between the farmer and all of the households receiving milk
- Milk should be from a single farm and not co-mingled

Key points

- The Michigan Department of Agriculture and Rural Development (MDARD) does not license or inspect the herd share portion of a dairy farm.
- Herd share programs are considered to include only FUW milk intended to be consumed by people.
- FUW milk is not for sale or resale.
- FUW milk cannot be distributed from a licensed food establishment.

Report of Michigan Fresh Unprocessed Whole Milk Workgroup

- Products such as butter, yogurt, cheeses, etc., made from FUW milk were not included in the Workgroup's discussions and are not considered by MDARD to be part of a herd share operation and therefore are subject to applicable MDARD laws and regulations.
- Advertising of herd shares is not regulated by MDARD.

The Workgroup felt comfortable with these decisions based on the fact that there is a defined consumer pool, rapid trace back is possible, and the farmer and shareholder are both responsible for maintaining the quality of the milk.

Report of Michigan Fresh Unprocessed Whole Milk Workgroup

AFTERWORD

by Pete Kennedy, Esq.

The Michigan Workgroup, which wrote the *Report on Fresh Unprocessed Whole Milk Workgroup*, consisted of regulators, academicians, a member of the dairy industry, and raw milk producers and consumers. This level of cooperation between groups with divergent views on raw milk has not occurred before, or since. If there was a single reason why the Michigan Workgroup was able to forge a consensus on raw milk, that would be the late Dr. Ted Beals, MD, the principal author of the Report.

Raw milk opponents and their experts often criticized evidence brought by those supporting its consumption as unscientific and anecdotal, but it is more difficult for them to raise that argument against Dr. Beals, a medical doctor. He had a CV that was over 100 pages long, which included training in microbiology, epidemiology and pathology – in addition to his certification as a medical doctor. Dr. Beals taught courses in pathology to University of Michigan graduate and medical students for over 30 years; he finished his career by serving as the national director of Pathology and Laboratory Services in the Department of Veterans Affairs, having oversight and responsibility for some 700 labs in the VA system.

He had also collected the largest database on foodborne illness outbreaks attributed to raw milk consumption, spanning 1999[1] to 2019. He found that the raw milk illnesses in his database were so few in number that it wasn't possible to establish any pattern on what caused illness from consuming the product.

Dr. Beals was one of the most important figures in the movement to expand raw milk legalization and access in the U.S. and Canada. He served as an expert witness before courts, legislature, and government agencies; presented on raw milk science and safety as a speaker and educator; and provided insight as a valued consultant for raw milk farmers in Michigan who had questions about their dairy operations. Dr. Beals worked directly and indirectly with farmers accused by the government of producing adulterated raw milk, never turning down a request for help. If there was a flaw in the government investigation or evidence exonerating the dairy farmer against charges of producing unsanitary milk, or making people sick, Dr. Beals would find it. If the producer was responsible for producing adulterated milk, he would suggest a way for the farmer to produce a safer product.

Report of Michigan Fresh Unprocessed Whole Milk Workgroup

Dr. Beals was the best expert witness the raw milk movement has had. He was a key witness in an Ontario court for farmer Michael Schmidt's successful defense of the legality of his herd share program, a case where a judge made the landmark ruling that there was a legal distinction between the public and private distribution of food, and that informed consumers had the right to waive the protection of the public health laws.[2] He was a formidable opponent for any state attorney trying to question him.

Aside from the Report, Dr. Beals and his late wife, Peggy Beals, RN, were the driving force behind two important books published by the nonprofit Farm-to-Consumer Foundation on the production of raw cow milk and raw goat milk. He also worked with his wife on her consumer guide to safe handling of raw milk, *Caring for Fresh Milk Consumers' Guide*,[3] a publication that has thousands of copies in circulation and is more timely than ever with the skyrocketing demand for raw milk.

Dr. Beals worked until nearly the end of his life; the last article he wrote included a comparison of milk samples from licensed raw milk dairies versus milk samples from dairies producing milk for pasteurization. He had accumulated and analyzed thousands of state-collected data on raw milk test results for pathogens from around the country, convincingly showing that the positive pathogen rate for milk samples from licensed raw milk dairies was extremely low, and much lower than for dairies producing milk for pasteurization.[4]

His final work provided strong proof for a contention that he and others in the raw milk movement had long made: that there are two raw milks, one for direct consumption and one for pasteurization.

Dr. Beals was largely responsible for building the consensus that resulted in the Workgroup report. He took the draft of the Report word by word, making sure he had agreement among the Workgroup members on everything he wrote.

There would be no opportunity for anyone in the Workgroup opposed to raw milk consumption to dissent from any of the Report's findings. The Report is a testament to the possibility of what can happen in the advancement of the science on raw milk risks and benefits if people working on the project understand one basic fact: people have the right to consume raw milk (consumption of raw milk has always been legal in all 50 states) and then provide the public with accurate information for each individual making a decision on whether to consume the product.

Report of Michigan Fresh Unprocessed Whole Milk Workgroup

The clash of cultures between anti-raw milk and pro-raw milk factions that existed in 2007 when the Michigan Workgroup began meeting, is still around today. A major difference today is that the tremendous growth in demand for raw milk has made it difficult for the anti-raw milk faction to curb access as much as it had been able to do in the past; the demand for raw milk has gone up almost without interruption for the past 20 years, but it has never been greater than it is today. The Make America Healthy Again (MAHA) movement and the realization by millions after COVID that they need to take charge of their own health, primarily through diet, is the reason for the current demand. Nevertheless, the anti-raw milk faction—instead of acknowledging that raw milk is here to stay and recognizing that it has a place in the market—continues to take the same actions it has been taking all along, in an attempt to reduce the supply and demand, including:

- Media broadcasting far and wide when a raw milk dairy has been shut down for a positive pathogen test, then remaining silent when the dairy is reinstated.

- Public health agencies investigating a foodborne illness outbreak stop looking for other potential causes once it finds out that some of the people sickened consumed raw milk.

- The media reporting nationally for days on a foodborne illness outbreak attributed to raw milk consumption, but reporting only once if a foodborne illness outbreak is blamed on pasteurized milk.

- Manipulating data on raw milk-linked illnesses to create a climate of fear to dissuade the public from consuming the product, aided by various alphabet-soup health agencies, and organizations (e.g., FDA, CDC, AMA, AAP, etc.) having their credentialed experts reinforce each other's opinion on how dangerous is raw milk.

- In 2024-2025, shutting down raw milk dairies for weeks at a time over questionable positive tests for Highly Pathogenic Avian Influenza (HPAI) when there isn't a shred of evidence that HPAI in any food has ever made anybody sick.[5]

One caveat: even though the federal regulation banning raw milk and raw milk products (other than raw cheese aged 60 days) in interstate commerce has been about as successful as alcohol Prohibition, lifting the ban could have the unintended consequence of restricting access; FDA could issue restrictive regulations with a high cost of compliance and then pressure states to adopt the

Report of Michigan Fresh Unprocessed Whole Milk Workgroup

same laws. A former dairy division director of FDA once said, "Drinking raw milk is like playing Russian roulette with your health"[6] and "raw milk is inherently dangerous and should not be consumed by anyone, at any time, for any reason"[7]. The evidence indicates that some people within FDA today still hold those views. FDA's harassment of raw cheese producers, chronicled in Catherine Donnelly's book (*Ending the War on Artisan Cheese*[8]), serves as a warning against repealing the interstate ban before there is a change in culture at FDA on raw dairy.

A start to changing the culture at FDA would be for the agency to acknowledge the peer-reviewed publications describing the benefits and safety of raw milk consumption, such as the Parsifal[9,10], Gabriel[11], Amish[12], and Whitehead/Lake[13] studies, as well as studies on the microbiome and, of course, the Michigan Workgroup report.

Health and Human Services Secretary (HHS), Robert F. Kennedy Jr., has stated that he wants to increase access to raw milk. He has also said that he wants to reestablish gold-standard science at HHS.[14]

How about launching an HHS-funded study on the role of raw milk in preventing chronic disease? Raw milk, along with beef and eggs, are arguably three of the most nutritious foods historically consumed by the majority of Americans; and these are foods most under attack from regulators and the scientific community.

Reversing the epidemic of chronic disease is a top priority of the new administration under Trump; raw milk can serve as a key component of that initiative. FDA should honor freedom of choice and recognize the fact that there are currently an estimated 15 to 20 million people drinking raw milk, and their fearmongering campaign against the product isn't changing their minds.

FDA can acknowledge the reality of the situation by taking any of the following actions:

- Posting peer-reviewed articles about raw milk's health benefits on its website;

- Publishing information from scientific journals for consumers about raw milk safe handling on the FDA website; Peg Beal's book, *Caring for Fresh Milk Consumers' Guide*[15], could be used as a resource.

- Submitting testimony in support of state legislation either legalizing or expanding raw milk sales. FDA used to submit testimony opposing state raw milk bills;

- Discontinuing policies or rules that condition a state's funding from, or rating with, the federal government on its raw milk laws;

- Amending the Pasteurized Milk Ordinance (PMO) (the federal document governing the production and distribution of raw milk for pasteurization), so that there is no longer a provision in it requiring that only pasteurized milk be sold to the final consumer.

As of early 2025, there are now 40 states that, by law or policy, allow the sale or distribution of raw milk for human consumption. In many of these states, the law limits access for the consumer. There currently aren't enough raw milk farmers, cows, or available land to meet the growing demand; the regulatory climate at the state, and especially the federal level, needs to improve. This development won't take place unless the culture against raw milk at FDA changes.

With the rise of the MAHA movement, there is an opportunity to expand on the work of Dr. Beals and the Michigan Workgroup and forge a national consensus that raw milk is a safe nutrient-dense food to which everyone should have access. Many have noted that mandatory pasteurization laws, more than any other factor, depleted the countryside of small farms and local wealth. Raw milk can be a centerpiece not only of a healthy revival, but also of a revival of rural life.

Report of Michigan Fresh Unprocessed Whole Milk Workgroup

REFERENCES

[1] Sally Fallon Morell. (2016). Raw Milk Safety: A Summary. *Wise Traditions Journal*, 17:4 (Winter 2016), p. 81. *https://www.westonaprice.org/wp-content/uploads/Winter-2016s.pdf*

[2] Pete Kennedy. (2010). Minnesota: MDA Considering Criminal Prosecution of Consumer. Farm-to-Consumer Legal Defense Fund. December 28, 2010. https://www.farmtoconsumer.org/blog/2010/12/28/minnesota-mda-considering-criminal-prosecution-of-consumer/

[3] Peggy Beals. (2011). Safe Handling - Consumers' Guide - Preserving the Quality of Fresh, Unprocessed Whole Milk, 4th edition. Spring House Press LLC. https://gianacliscaldwell.com/2011/10/08/must-have-booklet-for-consumers-and-sellers-of-raw-milk/

[4] Ted F. Beals. (2022). Observations on Fresh Unprocessed Milk Samples from States Regulating Dairies: There Are Two Kinds of Milk. Real Milk. January 23, 2022. *https://www.realmilk.com/observations-on-fresh-unprocessed-milk-samples/*

[5] Coleman, ME. (2024). Where Is the Evidence? Coleman Scientific Consulting. April 10, 2024. https://www.colemanscientific.org/blog/2024/4/7/where-is-the-evidence

[6] John F. Sheehan. (2005). Safety of Raw Milk On The Safety of Raw Milk (with a word about (with a word about pasteurization). FDA/CFSAN Division of Dairy and Egg Safety. (PowerPoint slides). *https://www.fda.gov/media/119007/download*

[7] Clash Over Unpasteurized Milk Gets Raw. (2008?). Marler Clark the Food Safety Law Firm. (Blog). *https://marlerclark.com/media_relations/a-clash-over-unpasteurized-milk-gets-raw*

[8] Catherine W. Donnelly. (2019). Ending the War on Artisan Cheese: The Inside Story of Government Overreach and the Struggle to Save Traditional Raw Milk Cheesemakers. (Paperback). White River Junction, Vermont: Chelsea Green Publishing.

[9] Alfvén T, Braun-Fahrländer C, Brunekreef B, von Mutius E, Riedler J, Scheynius A, van Hage M, Wickman M, Benz MR, Budde J, Michels KB, Schram D, Ublagger E, Waser M, Pershagen G; PARSIFAL study group. (2006). Allergic diseases and atopic sensitization in children related to farming and

anthroposophic lifestyle--the PARSIFAL study. Allergy. 2006 Apr;61(4):414-21. doi: 10.1111/j.1398-9995.2005.00939.x. PMID: 16512802. https://pubmed.ncbi.nlm.nih.gov/16512802/

[10] Waser M, Michels KB, Bieli C, Flöistrup H, Pershagen G, von Mutius E, Ege M, Riedler J, Schram-Bijkerk D, Brunekreef B, van Hage M, Lauener R, Braun-Fahrländer C; PARSIFAL Study team. (2007). Inverse association of farm milk consumption with asthma and allergy in rural and suburban populations across Europe. Clin Exp Allergy. 2007 May;37(5):661-70. doi: 10.1111/j.1365-2222.2006.02640.x. PMID: 17456213. https://pubmed.ncbi.nlm.nih.gov/17456213/

[11] Loss G, Apprich S, Waser M, Kneifel W, Genuneit J, Büchele G, Weber J, Sozanska B, Danielewicz H, Horak E, van Neerven RJ, Heederik D, Lorenzen PC, von Mutius E, Braun-Fahrländer C; GABRIELA study group. (2011). The protective effect of farm milk consumption on childhood asthma and atopy: the GABRIELA study. J Allergy Clin Immunol. 2011 Oct;128(4):766-773.e4. doi: 10.1016/j.jaci.2011.07.048. Epub 2011 Aug 27. PMID: 21875744. https://pubmed.ncbi.nlm.nih.gov/21875744/

[12] Vercelli D. (2023). From Amish farm dust to bacterial lysates: The long and winding road to protection from allergic disease. Semin Immunol. 2023 Jul;68:101779. doi: 10.1016/j.smim.2023.101779. Epub 2023 May 19. PMID: 37210851; PMCID: PMC10330614. *https://pmc.ncbi.nlm.nih.gov/articles/PMC10330614/*

[13] Whitehead J, Lake B. (2018). Recent Trends in Unpasteurized Fluid Milk Outbreaks, Legalization, and Consumption in the United States. PLoS Curr. 2018 Sep 13;10:ecurrents.outbreaks.bae5a0fd685616839c9cf857792730d1. doi: 10.1371/currents.outbreaks.bae5a0fd685616839c9cf857792730d1. PMID: 30279996; PMCID: PMC6140832. https://pubmed.ncbi.nlm.nih.gov/30279996/

[14] FDA News Release. (2025, April 11). FDA Honored to Welcome HHS Secretary Robert F. Kennedy, Jr. to FDA Campus. https://www.fda.gov/news-events/press-announcements/fda-honored-welcome-hhs-secretary-robert-f-kennedy-jr-fda-campus

[15] Peggy Beals. (2016). Caring for Fresh Milk Consumers' Guide – Consumers' Guide – Preserving the Quality of Fresh, Unprocessed Whole Milk, 5th edition. The Weston A. Price Foundation, pub.

CITED REFERENCES

Alfvén, T., Braun-Fahrländer, C., Brunekreef, B., von Mutius, E., Riedler, J., Scheynius, A., van Hage, M., Wickman, M., Benz, M. R., Budde, J., Michels, K. B., Schram, D., Ublagger, E., Waser, M., Pershagen, G., & PARSIFAL study group. (2006). Allergic diseases and atopic sensitization in children related to farming and anthroposophic lifestyle--the PARSIFAL study. *Allergy, 61*(4), 414–421. https://doi.org/10.1111/j.1398-9995.2005.00939.x

American Association of Medical Milk Commissions. (1912). *Sixth annual meeting of the American Association of Medical Milk Commissions.* Proctor & Collier Press. https://books.google.com/books?id=cqYDAAAAYAAJ&dq=+henry+coit+certified+milk+movement&source=gbs summarys&cad=O

Bach, S.J., McAllister, T.A., Veira, D. M., Gannon, V.P.J., & Holley, R.A. (2002). Transmission and control of escherichia coli O157:H7—A review. *Canadian Journal of Animal Science, 82*(4), 475-490. https://doi.org/10.4141/A02-021

Baker, D.R., Moxley, R.A., Steele, M.B., LeJeune, J.T., Christopher-Hennings, J., Chen, D., Hardwidge, P.R., & Francis, D.H. (2007). Differences in virulence among escherichia coli O157:H7 strains isolated from humans during disease outbreaks and from healthy cattle. *Appl Environ Microbiol 73,* 1-14. https://doi.org/10.1128/AEM.00755-07

Beals, P. (2016). *Caring for fresh milk consumers' guide – consumers' guide – preserving the quality of fresh, unprocessed whole milk,* 5th edition. Washington, DC: The Weston A. Price Foundation, pub.

Beals, P. (2011). *Safe handling: consumers' guide to fresh, unprocessed whole milk,* 4th edition. Spring House Press LLC.

Beals, T.F. (2022, Jan 23). Observations on fresh unprocessed milk samples from states regulating dairies: there are two kinds of milk. [Blog post]. *Real Milk. https://www.realmilk.com/observations-on-fresh-unprocessed-milk-samples/*

Beals, T.F. (2008, Mar 29). Pilot survey of cow share consumer/owners lactose intolerance section. [Blog post]. *RealMilk.com.* https://www.realmilk.com/lactose-intolerance-survey/

Beals, T.F. (2011). *Those pathogens - what you should know.* [PowerPoint slides]. Third International Raw Milk Symposium. Retrieved April 11, 2025, from https://www.realmilk.com/wp-content/uploads/2012/11/2011_Raw_Milk_Symposium_-_Beals.pdf

Bronzwaer, S., Hugas, M., Collins, J. D., Newell, D. G., Robinson, T., Mäkelä, P., & Havelaar, A. (2009). EFSA's 12th scientific colloquium--assessing health benefits of controlling campylobacter in the food chain. *International Journal of Food Microbiology, 131*(2-3), 284–285. https://doi.org/10.1016/j.ijfoodmicro.2009.01.033

Centers for Disease Control and Prevention (CDC). (2007). *Foodborne diseases active surveillance network (FoodNet) population survey atlas of exposures, 2006-2007.* Atlanta, Georgia: U.S. Department of Health and Human Services, Centers for Disease Control and Prevention, Corporate Authors(s) : National Center for Zoonotic, Vector-Borne, and Enteric Diseases (U.S.). Division of Foodborne, Bacterial, and Mycotic Diseases. Enteric Diseases Epidemiology Branch. Retrieved April 11, 2025, from https://stacks.cdc.gov/view/cdc/24453

Coleman, ME. (2024, Apr10). Where is the evidence? [Blog post]. *Coleman Scientific Consulting.* https://www.colemanscientific.org/blog/2024/4/7/where-is-the-evidence

Committee on the Review of the Use of Scientific Criteria and Performance Standards for Safe Food. (2003). *Scientific criteria to ensure safe food.* [Chapter 1: Historical perspective on the use of food safety criteria and performance standards.] Washington, DC: The National Academies Press. https://doi.org/10.17226/10690. Cited url: http://books.nap.edu/openbook.php?record id=10690&page=13 [Redirected to: https://nap.nationalacademies.org/read/10690/chapter/3]

Czaplicki, A. (2007). Pure milk is better than purified milk: pasteurization and milk purity in Chicago, 1908-1916. *Social Science History 31*(3), 411-433. doi:10.1017/S0145553200013808. https://muse.jhu.edu/article/220538.

Desch, K., & Motto, D. (2007). Is there a shared pathophysiology for thrombotic thrombocytopenic purpura and hemolytic-uremic syndrome?. *Journal of the American Society of Nephrology, 18*(9), 2457–2460. https://doi.org/10.1681/ASN.2007010062

Donnelly, C.W. (2019). *Ending the war on artisan cheese: the inside story of government overreach and the struggle to save traditional raw milk cheesemakers.* [Paperback]. White River Junction, Vermont: Chelsea Green Publishing.

Douglas II, W.C. (2007). *The raw truth about milk* (formerly, *The milk book,* 1984). [Chapter IV: Udder Propaganda]. Panama: Rhino Publishing, S.A. Retrieved April 10, 2025, from https://ia801203.us.archive.org/11/items/The_Raw_Truth_About_Milk/The_Raw_Truth_About_Milk.pdf

Doyle, M. P., & Roman, D. J. (1982). Prevalence and survival of campylobacter jejuni in unpasteurized milk. *Applied and Environmental Microbiology, 44*(5), 1154–1158. https://doi.org/10.1128/aem.44.5.1154-1158.1982

Dupuis, E.M. (2002). *Nature's perfect food: how milk became America's drink.* New York, NY: New York University Press. Obtain from https://nyupress.org/9780814719381/natures-perfect-food/

Elwood, P. C., Pickering, J. E., & Fehily, A. M. (2007). Milk and dairy consumption, diabetes and the metabolic syndrome: the Caerphilly prospective study. *Journal of Epidemiology and Community Health, 61*(8), 695–698. https://doi.org/10.1136/jech.2006.053157

Fallon Morell, S. (2016). Raw milk safety: A summary. [PowerPoint slides]. *Wise Traditions Journal, 17*(4), 81. *https://www.westonaprice.org/wp-content/uploads/Winter-2016s.pdf*

Fallon Morell, S. (2024). *The safety and health benefits of raw milk.*[PowerPoint slides]. A Campaign for Real Milk. Retrieved April 10, 2025, from https://www.realmilk.com/real-milk-powerpoint/

Fankhauser, D.B. (1999, Nov 22). Comparison of nutritional content of various milks. [Blog post]. *David Fankhauser.* University of Cincinnati Clermont College, Cincinnati, Ohio. Cited url: http://biology.clc.uc.edu/fankhauser/Cheese/milk_content.htm [Revised url: https://fankhauserblog.wordpress.com/tag/microbiology/page/3/]

Farm-to-Consumer Legal Defense Fund. (2012, Apr 4). Judge dismisses FDA raw milk lawsuit. [Blog post]. https://www.farmtoconsumer.org/blog/2012/04/04/judge-dismisses-fda-raw-milk-lawsuit-2/

Food and Drug Administration. (2012). *Bad bug book, foodborne pathogenic microorganisms and natural toxins*, Second Edition. [Cited url: https://www.fda.gov/food/foodsafety/foodborneillness/foodborneillnessfoodbornepathgensnaturaltoxins/badbugbook/ucm070064.htm Revised url: https://www.fda.gov/food/foodborne-pathogens/bad-bug-book-second-edition]

Food and Drug Administration. (2025, April 11). FDA honored to welcome HHS secretary Robert F. Kennedy, Jr. to FDA campus. FDA News Release. https://www.fda.gov/news-events/press-announcements/fda-honored-welcome-hhs-secretary-robert-f-kennedy-jr-fda-campus

Food and Drug Administration. (2005). Food and drug administration milestones in U.S. food and drug law history. (Website). Current as of 1/30/2023. Cited url: http://www.fda.gov/opacom/backgrounders/miles.html [Revised url: https://www.fda.gov/about-fda/fda-history/milestones-us-food-and-drug-law]

Fox, P.F., & Kelly, A.L. (2006). Indigenous enzymes in milk: overview and historical aspects - part 1. *International Dairy Journal 16*(6), 500-516. https://doi.org/10.1016/j.idairyj.2005.09.013

Fox, P.F., & Kelly, A.L. (2006). "Indigenous enzymes in milk: overview and historical aspects - part 2. *International Dairy Journal 16*(6), 517-532. https://doi.org/10.1016/j.idairyj.2005.09.017

Gillespie, I., & McLauchlin, J. (2008). Advisory committee on the microbiological safety of food update listeriosis in England and Wales. Health Protection Agency Centre for Infections. ACM/879, December 2007. Retrieved May 2, 2025, from https://acmsf.food.gov.uk/sites/default/files/mnt/drupal_data/sources/files/multimedia/pdfs/committee/879listeria.pdf

Goff, D., Hill, A., & Ferrer, M.A. (1996). *Dairy chemistry and physics.* [Dairy Science and Technology eBook]. Toronto, Canada: University of Guelph. Cited url: http://www.foodsci.uoguelph.ca/dairyedu/chem.html [Revised url, ebook: https://books.lib.uoguelph.ca/dairyscienceandtechnologyebook/]

Gould, L.H., Bopp, C., Strockbine, N., Atkinson, R., Baselski, V., Body, B., Carey, R., Crandall, C., Hurd, S., Kaplan, R., Neill, M., Shea, S., Somsel, P., Tobin-D'Angelo, M., Griffin, P.M., Gerner-Smidt, P., & Centers for Disease Control and Prevention (CDC). (2009). Recommendations for diagnosis of shiga toxin--producing escherichia coli infections by clinical laboratories. *MMWR. Recommendations and reports : Morbidity and mortality weekly report. Recommendations and reports, 58*(RR-12), 1–14. https://pubmed.ncbi.nlm.nih.gov/19834454/

Grohman, J.S. (2003). *Keeping a family cow*. Dixfield, ME: Coburn Press.

Haug, A., Høstmark, A. T., & Harstad, O. M. (2007). Bovine milk in human nutrition--a review. *Lipids in Health and Disease, 6*, 25. https://doi.org/10.1186/1476-511X-6-25. https://pubmed.ncbi.nlm.nih.gov/17894873/ [Cited url: http://www.pubmedcentral.nih.gov/articlerender.fcgi?artid=2039733 Revised url, for Table 1: https://lipidworld.biomedcentral.com/articles/10.1186/1476-511X-6-25/tables/1]

Husu, J.R. (1990). Epidemiological studies on the occurrence of listeria monocytogenes in the feces of dairy cattle. *Journal of Veterinary Medicine, Series B*, 37(1-10), 276-282. https://doi.org/10.1111/j.1439-0450.1990.tb01059.x

Inglis, G. D., Kalischuk, L. D., & Busz, H. W. (2004). Chronic shedding of campylobacter species in beef cattle. *Journal of Applied Microbiology, 97*(2), 410-420. https://doi.org/10.1111/j.1365-2672.2004.02313.x

Ivanek, R., Gröhn, Y. T., & Wiedmann, M. (2006). Listeria monocytogenes in multiple habitats and host populations: review of available data for mathematical modeling. *Foodborne Pathogens and Disease, 3*(4), 319–336. https://doi.org/10.1089/fpd.2006.3.319

Kennedy, P. (2017, Aug 30). Michigan raw dairy – how one consumer made an impact. [Blog post]. *RealMilk.com*. https://www.realmilk.com/michigan-raw-dairy-one-consumer-made-impact/

Kennedy, P. (2010, Dec 28). Minnesota: MDA considering criminal prosecution of consumer. [Blog post]. *Farm-to-Consumer Legal Defense Fund*. https://www.farmtoconsumer.org/blog/2010/12/28/minnesota-mda-considering-criminal-prosecution-of-consumer/

Kennedy, P. (2022, Nov 22). Solari food series: raw milk nation. [Blog post]. *The Solari Report*. https://home.solari.com/solari-food-series-raw-milk-nation/

Kothary, M., & Babu, U. (2001). Infective dose of foodborne pathogens in volunteers: a review. *Journal of Food Safety 21*(1), 49-73. https://onlinelibrary.wiley.com/doi/abs/10.1111/j.1745-4565.2001.tb00307.x

Loss, G., Apprich, S., Waser, M., Kneifel, W., Genuneit, J., Büchele, G., Weber, J., Sozanska, B., Danielewicz, H., Horak, E., van Neerven, R. J., Heederik, D., Lorenzen, P. C., von Mutius, E., Braun-Fahrländer, C., & GABRIELA study group. (2011). The protective effect of farm milk consumption on childhood asthma and atopy: the GABRIELA study. *The Journal of Allergy and Clinical Immunology, 128*(4), 766–773.e4. https://doi.org/10.1016/j.jaci.2011.07.048

Manning, S.D., Motiwala, A.S., Springman, A.C., Qi, W., Lacher, D.W., Ouellette, L.M., Mladonicky, J.M., Somsel, P., Rudrik, J.T., Dietrich, S.E., Zhang, W., Swaminathan, B., Alland, D., & Whittam, T.S. (2008). Variation in virulence among clades of escherichia coli O157:H7 associated with disease outbreaks. *Proc. Natl. Acad. Sci. U.S.A. 105*(12), 4868-4873. https://doi.org/10.1073/pnas.0710834105

Marler Clark the Food Safety Law Firm. (circa 2008). Clash over unpasteurized milk gets raw. (Blog). https://marlerclark.com/media_relations/a-clash-over-unpasteurized-milk-gets-raw

Massa, S., Goffredo, E., Altieri, C., & Natola, K. (1999). Fate of escherichia coli O157:H7 in unpasteurized milk stored at 8 degrees c. *Letters in Applied Microbiology, 28*(1), 89–92. https://doi.org/10.1046/j.1365-2672.1999.00408.x

McGee, H. (2004). *On food and cooking: The science and lore of the kitchen.* [Chapter 1: Milk and dairy products]. New York, NY: Scribner. http://www.curiouscook.com

National Conference on Interstate Milk Shipments. (2009). *History and accomplishments of the national conference on interstate milk shipments, 2009 Edition* [p. 47 for 2001 entry]. NCIMS, 123 Buena Vista Drive, Frankfort, KY 40601. Cited url: http://www.ncims.org [Revision, 2009 ed.: https://ncims.org/wp-content/uploads/2018/10/History-and-Accomplishments-of-the-NCIMS-through-2009.pdf]

The National Dairy Council. (2006). Milk's unique nutrient package'. [Poster]. https://ansc.umd.edu/sites/ansc.umd.edu/files/files/documents/Extension/Milks-Nutrient-Package.pdf

NICHD, author. (2006). Building strong bones: calcium information for health care providers. U.S. Department of Health and Human Services - National

Institute of Child Health and Human Development. [17.09.2014]. In NIH Publication No 05-5305. https://www.nichd.nih.gov/publications/pubs/documents/NICHD_MM_HC_FS_rev.pdf. [Google Scholar]

Oberleas, D., & Prasad, A. S. (1969). Adequacy of trace minerals in bovine milk for human consumption. *The American journal of clinical nutrition, 22*(2), 196–199. https://doi.org/10.1093/ajcn/22.2.196

Oliver, H.F., Wiedmann, M., Boor, K.J. (2007). Environmental reservoir and transmission into the mammalian host. In: Goldfine, H., Shen, H. (eds) *Listeria monocytogenes: Pathogenesis and Host Response*. Springer, Boston, MA. https://doi.org/10.1007/978-0-387-49376-3_6

Patton, C. M., Nicholson, M. A., Ostroff, S. M., Ries, A. A., Wachsmuth, I. K., & Tauxe, R. V. (1993). Common somatic o and heat-labile serotypes among campylobacter strains from sporadic infections in the United States. *Journal of Clinical Microbiology, 31*(6), 1525–1530. https://doi.org/10.1128/jcm.31.6.1525-1530.1993

Patton, S. (2004). *Milk its remarkable contribution to human health and well-being*. Piscataway, NJ: Transaction Publisher.

Patton S. (1999). Some practical implications of the milk mucins. *Journal of Dairy Science, 82*(6), 1115–1117. https://doi.org/10.3168/jds.S0022-0302(99)75334-8

Perkin M. R. (2007). Unpasteurized milk: health or hazard?. *Clinical and Experimental Allergy : Journal of the British Society for Allergy and Clinical Immunology, 37*(5), 627–630. https://doi.org/10.1111/j.1365-2222.2007.02715.x

Perkin, M. R., & Strachan, D. P. (2006). Which aspects of the farming lifestyle explain the inverse association with childhood allergy?. *The Journal of Allergy and Clinical Immunology, 117*(6), 1374–1381. https://doi.org/10.1016/j.jaci.2006.03.008

Potter, R. C., Kaneene, J. B., & Hall, W. N. (2003). Risk factors for sporadic campylobacter jejuni infections in rural Michigan: a prospective case-control study. *American Journal of Public Health, 93*(12), 2118–2123. https://doi.org/10.2105/ajph.93.12.2118

Public Health Service/Food and Drug Administration. (2007). *Grade "A" pasteurized milk ordinance, including provisions from the grade "A" condensed and dry milk products and condensed and dry whey--supplement I to the grade "A" pasteurized milk ordinance*. [Cited url: http://www.michigan.gov/documents/mda/MDA_DP_07PMOFinal_251324_7.pdf Revised url, 2017 ed.: https://www.michigan.gov/mdard/-/media/Project/Websites/mdard/documents/food-dairy/dairy/grade_a_pasteurized_milk_ordinance.pdf]

Scallan, E., Hoekstra, R. M., Angulo, F. J., Tauxe, R. V., Widdowson, M. A., Roy, S. L., Jones, J. L., & Griffin, P. M. (2011). Foodborne illness acquired in the United States--major pathogens. *Emerging Infectious Diseases, 17*(1), 7–15. https://doi.org/10.3201/eid1701.p11101

Schmid, R. (2003). *Untold story of milk: green pastures, contented cows and raw dairy products*. Wash., DC: New Trends Publishing. [Note: Revised and Updated in 2009]

Semenov, A.V. (2008). Ecology and modeling of escherichia coli O157:H7 and salmonella enterica serovars typhimurium in cattle manure and soils. [Doctoral thesis]. Wageningen University, Netherlands: Biological Farming Systems Group. https://edepot.wur.nl/122071

Sheehan, J.F. (2005). Safety of raw milk on the safety of raw milk (with a word about pasteurization). [PowerPoint slides]. FDA/CFSAN Division of Dairy and Egg Safety. https://www.fda.gov/media/119007/download

Thomson, J.C. (1943). Pasteurised milk, a national menace. *The Kingston Chronicle*. Edinburgh, Scotland. Retrieved April 10, 2025 from https://www.seleneriverpress.com/images/pdfs/Pasteurised_Milk_-_a_National_Menace_-_Scotland_-_JC_THOMSON_1943__Reprint_28C.pdf

Uzzau, S., Brown, D. J., Wallis, T., Rubino, S., Leori, G., Bernard, S., Casadesús, J., Platt, D. J., & Olsen, J. E. (2000). Host adapted serotypes of salmonella enterica. *Epidemiology and Infection, 125*(2), 229–255. https://doi.org/10.1017/s0950268899004379

Van Loon, D. (1976). *The family cow*. North Adams, MA: Storey Publishing, LLC.

Vercelli, D. (2023). From Amish farm dust to bacterial lysates: the long and winding road to protection from allergic disease. *Seminars in Immunology, 68*, 101779. https://doi.org/10.1016/j.smim.2023.101779

Wagenaar, J. A., Mevius, D. J., & Havelaar, A. H. (2006). Campylobacter in primary animal production and control strategies to reduce the burden of human campylobacteriosis. *Revue Scientifique et Technique (International Office of Epizootics), 25*(2), 581–594.

Walstra, P., Walstra, P., Wouters, J.T.M., & Geurts, T.J. (2005). *Dairy Science and Technology* (2nd ed.). [eBook]. CRC Press. https://doi.org/10.1201/9781420028010

Ward, R. E., & German, J. B. (2004). Understanding milk's bioactive components: a goal for the genomics toolbox. *The Journal of Nutrition, 134*(4), 962S–7S. https://doi.org/10.1093/jn/134.4.962S

Waser, M., Michels, K. B., Bieli, C., Flöistrup, H., Pershagen, G., von Mutius, E., Ege, M., Riedler, J., Schram-Bijkerk, D., Brunekreef, B., van Hage, M., Lauener, R., Braun-Fahrländer, C., & PARSIFAL Study team (2007). Inverse association of farm milk consumption with asthma and allergy in rural and suburban populations across Europe. *Clinical and Experimental Allergy : Journal of the British Society for Allergy and Clinical Immunology, 37*(5), 661–670. https://doi.org/10.1111/j.1365-2222.2006.02640.x

Waserman M. J. (1972). Henry L. Coit and the Certified Milk Movement in the Development of Modern Pediatrics. *Bulletin of the history of medicine, 46*(4), 359–390. Cited url: http://www.ncbi.nlm.nih.gov/pubmed/4562983 [Redirected to: https://pubmed.ncbi.nlm.nih.gov/4562983/]

Weston A. Price Foundation. (2012, March 4). Rebuttal to the testimony of John F. Sheehan. [Blog post]. Retrieved April 10, 2025, from https://www.realmilk.com/wp-content/uploads/2000/01/ResponsetoJohnSheehanTestimony.pdf

Weston A. Price Foundation. (2006, Oct 27). Action against raw milk in Michigan and Indiana. [Blog post]. https://www.westonaprice.org/action-against-raw-milk-in-michigan-and-indiana/#gsc.tab=0

Whitehead, J., & Lake, B. (2018). Recent trends in unpasteurized fluid milk outbreaks, legalization, and consumption in the United States. *PLoS*

Currents, 10, ecurrents.outbreaks.bae5a0fd685616839c9cf857792730d1. https://doi.org/10.1371/currents.outbreaks.bae5a0fd685616839c9cf857792730d1

Wiedmann M. (2002). Molecular subtyping methods for listeria monocytogenes. *Journal of AOAC International, 85*(2), 524–531. PMID: 11990041. https://pubmed.ncbi.nlm.nih.gov/11990041/

World Health Organization (WHO) and the Food and Agriculture Organization (FAO) of the United Nations (2004). Risk assessment of listeria monocytogenes in ready-to-eat foods—interpretative summary. *Microbiological Risk Assessment Series,* No. 4. Rome. https://www.fao.org/fileadmin/templates/agns/pdf/jemra/mra4_en.pdf

Yilmaz, T., Moyer, B., MacDonell, R.E., Cordero-Coma, M., & Gallagher, M.J. (2009). Outbreaks associated with unpasteurized milk and soft cheese: an overview of consumer safety. *Food Protection Trends 29*(4), 211-222. Retrieved May 2, 2025, from https://www.cdr.wisc.edu/assets/pipeline-pdfs/2.2-FPT-29-211-unpast-milk-cheese.pdf

Copyright © 2025 by Food Freedom Foundation

Foreword copyright © 2025 by Sally Fallon Morell

All rights reserved. No part of this book may be reproduced in any manner without the express written consent of the publisher, except in the case of brief excerpts in critical reviews or articles. All inquiries should be addressed to Skyhorse Publishing, 307 West 36th Street, 11th Floor, New York, NY 10018.

Skyhorse Publishing books may be purchased in bulk at special discounts for sales promotion, corporate gifts, fund-raising, or educational purposes. Special editions can also be created to specifications. For details, contact the Special Sales Department, Skyhorse Publishing, 307 West 36th Street, 11th Floor, New York, NY 10018 or info@skyhorsepublishing.com.

Skyhorse® and Skyhorse Publishing® are registered trademarks of Skyhorse Publishing, Inc.®, a Delaware corporation.

Visit our website at www.skyhorsepublishing.com.

10 9 8 7 6 5 4 3 2 1

Library of Congress Control Number: 2025937470

Cover design by David Ter-Avanesyan
Cover photo credit: Getty Images

Print ISBN: 978-1-5107-8495-6
Ebook ISBN: 978-1-5107-8496-3

Printed in the United States of America